Healing Massage Techniques

A Study of Eastern and Western Methods

Frances M. Tappan, B.S., M.A., Ed.D.

Reston Publishing Company, Inc.
A Prentice-Hall Company
Reston, Virginia

Library of Congress Cataloging in Publication Data

Tappan, Frances M
  Healing massage techniques.

  Bibliography: p. 252
  Includes index.
  1. Massage. 2. Acupuncture. I. Title.
RM721.T2178   615'.822   78-683
ISBN 0-8359-2821-7

Video tapes demonstrating *Healing Massage Techniques* will be available through the School of Allied Health Professions, Director of Communications and Media, University of Connecticut, Box U101, Storrs, Conn. 06268. All profit from rental or sale of these tapes will be donated to the Fran Tappan Student Aid Fund.

© 1978 by Reston Publishing Company, Inc.
A Prentice-Hall Company
Reston, Virginia 22090

10 9 8 7 6 5 4 3 2

Printed in the United States of America

Contents

Foreword

It has been my pleasure to meet and work with Dr. Tappan since 1975. During that time I have developed a great respect for her knowledge and skill. There is a need today for more emphasis on the true value of massage, particularly as it involves touching the patient, an art almost forgotten in the hustle of today's treatment techniques. A few minutes of massage can be of untold value in establishing a warm relationship with the patient. It can also acquaint the person giving the treatment with the exact nature of the disorders, which can be felt by trained and sensitive fingers.

To my knowledge, this is the first textbook on massage that compares Eastern massage techniques with methods practiced in the Western world. Although Eastern and Western medical philosophies differ in many ways, the similarities in their approaches to patient care are emphasized in this text, particularly as the effects of massage are related to blood flow, endocrine exchange, and the central nervous system.

Both Eastern and Western medicine are actively researching endorphins and enkephalins for relief of pain. Dr. Tappan's text includes a careful research of contemporary physiological explanations for relief of pain by the use of massage, especially the use of finger pressure to acupuncture points and the correlation between the overlapping areas of Bindegewebsmassage and acupuncture points.

This book is certainly most contemporary and inclusive of practically every known method of massage. I consider it a great contribution to all fields of all medicine that use massage as a part of patient care with a human touch.

JOSEPH YAO

Preface

This book describes the methods of massage brought together by the author based on courses taken and taught in the United States, Europe, and the Orient over the past 25 years. Its purpose is to present techniques that are clearly described and illustrated.

The massage systems of Albert J. Hoffa, Mary McMillan, James Cyriax, and James B. Mennell are discussed. Before the deaths of Dr. Mennell and Mary McMillan, the author was able to consult with them to assure the accuracy of the descriptions of the methods they used. Elisabeth Dicke's Bindegewebsmassage is discussed in more detail than in previous writings on this subject. The author studied these techniques at the Elisabeth Dicke School in Uberlingen, Germany and their descriptions were verified by Genette Elmiger, a Swiss woman who spoke English and German, and studied with Elisabeth Dicke before her death. Maria Ebner's text on connective tissue was also used extensively to clarify interpretations that were difficult to understand in the translation of *Meine Bindegewebsmassage.*

The author traveled to the Orient in 1975 to study acupuncture. Twenty acupuncture points are used in this book to illustrate how finger pressure can be incorporated into the massage routines for purposes of healing.

Subsequently the author studied Eunice Ingham's "Zone Therapy," often referred to as "reflexology." An overview of this system is also included in this text.

As a practice guide, cases are presented, including samples of many of the illnesses and injuries where massage can be usefully applied. This approach leads toward solving actual problems and recognizing that massage is only one aspect of the patient's total plan for care, since the legal, practical, and psychological aspects of each case must also be considered.

The illustrations showing the patterns of the massage strokes were made by applying fingerpaint to the hands of the masseur; the pattern left as one massages serves as a guide. Those who are learning can try to reproduce these same patterns with powder.

This book also presents the results of recent research in areas relevant to massage. For example, it has been recently discovered that massage may stimulate the release of endorphin. Reports of such findings are presented along with a discussion of the use of various biofeedback procedures. Through the use of sophisticated electronic equipment, these procedures assist both masseur and patient to see, hear, or feel the physiological changes that lead to homeostasis as an effect of massage.

Doctors Alyce and Elmer Green, at the Menninger Clinic in Topeka, Kansas, have done extensive research relating to the psychosomatic approach to medicine, emphasizing stress as the principal factor producing dysfunction and pathological change in the patient. Autogenic feedback training evokes changes opposite to those produced by stress and thus has importance for preventive medicine. Since one purpose of massage is relaxation and relief of stress, it will be doubly effective if the one doing the massage can provide autogenic phrases to increase the effectiveness of the massage.

Dolores Krieger has proven that touching, with a desire to heal, can actually increase hemoglobin. This too is discussed.

The emotional reactions to pain must be resolved before pain can be relieved. The extent to which pain can be relieved by massage combined with consideration of the patient's emotional state is included.

Acknowledgments

It would be humanly impossible to give adequate acknowledgment to all of the many fine people who have contributed to the writing of this book. Primary recognition should be given to Lucille Daniels, whose vision and wisdom assisted the author in building a solid foundation in the form of a Master's thesis on massage.

Josephine A. Dolan, Associate Professor, School of Nursing, University of Connecticut, gave valuable advice concerning the use of massage in the field of nursing.

The members of the staff of the School of Physical Therapy at the University of Connecticut who willingly gave their time, energy, and personal resources deserve credit for their valuable assistance, especially Vera Kaska, who used this material for two years and made worthwhile suggestions that made this text clearer to those using it for the first time.

Words cannot express my appreciation to the people who typed, drew the original sketches, and provided excellent editorial service, often working far into the night to meet the many deadlines involved in the production of this book, namly Gerri Pellecchia, Virginia Darrow, Nancy Wahnowsky, and Patricia McClellan Miller.

My thanks also to Dorothy McLaughlin, who was my patient and loyal companion as we studied acupuncture in Taipei, Taiwan, and to Dr. Min der Huang, our primary professor; to Dr. Edith Pao, who made it possible for us to study in Taiwan; and to Dr. Joseph Yao, Donald Courtial, and Dorothy McLaughlin for their assistance with descriptions and locations of the twenty acupuncture points used most commonly and thereby selected for study in this publication.

Part I

General Information

Chapter 1

Introduction

Massage is the systematic and scientific manipulation of the soft tissues of the body. Although massage can be applied by electrical equipment such as vibrators, rollers, or hydrotherapeutic turbines, the purpose of this text is to describe those techniques which can be applied by use of the hands. Regardless of the individual touch developed in massage, these manipulations will be gliding, percussing, compressing, or vibrating in nature.

TERMINOLOGY

An ancient Chinese book, *The Cong-Fou of the Tao-Tse*, of which a French translation appeared about a century ago, was probably the foundation both of our modern massage and of the manual Swedish movements, so admirably elaborated and systematized by Per Henrik Ling. Since the French brought Chinese massage to the West, most of the world continues to use the French terminology for massage strokes. Therefore, strokes which glide are called *effleurage*; those which knead are called *petrissage*; those which strike are called *tapotement*; those which compress are called *friction*; and those which shake or vibrate are called *vibration*.

PURPOSES OF MASSAGE

There are innumerable situations that cause a metabolic imbalance within the soft tissues. Most of these can be treated with massage. The purpose of massage is to bring about any of the physiological, mechanical, or psychological effects attributed to this type of treatment. Relaxation, relief from pain, reduction of certain types of edema, and increased range of motion can be accomplished through the use of massage. Massage is usually combined with other therapeutic measures, and often provides a form of passive exercise when stretching techniques are used.

Massage will not only physiologically relieve pain and metabolically prepare the injured or involved muscles for exercise to their fullest capacity, but it will also encourage the confidence of the patient. Moreover, the massage itself enables the operator to evaluate the patient's soft tissue much more effectively than any verbal or written report could.

In addition to the treatment of injured or ill people, massage can be used in athletics to ready healthy muscles for strenuous activity, or to assist the body in recovering from the aftereffects of such activity.

The Orientals teach massage to their children and feel very strongly that it is the responsibility of one human being to another to exchange such services. Dr. Katsusuke Serizawa, professor at the Tokyo University of Education, has written a book on massage promoting holistic treatment.[1] He is convinced that a return to caring treatment can help save mankind from the isolation and inhumanity of the modern condition.

In addition to the wide use of massage, acupuncture is practiced in all Oriental nations. Knowledge of acupuncture is useful in the practice of massage because finger compression on the acupuncture points can be very effective. Due to extensive recent publicity one might think that acupuncture is the *only* Oriental method of treatment for injury or illness. Nothing could be further from the truth. Mao Tse-tung and the Communist Party of China attached great importance to the development of Chinese medicine. In 1958, during the "Great Leap Forward," the combining of Chinese and Western medicine resulted in acupuncture anesthesia, marking a great advancement in the science of acupuncture. Acupuncture is only part of traditional Oriental medicine, which is founded on a philosophy of life dealing with the interaction

---

[1] Katsusuke Serizawa, *Massage, The Oriental Method,* 8th printing. San Francisco, Calif.: Japan Publications, Inc., 1974.

between the physician and the patient, the emotions of the person who is afflicted, and the stresses he experiences from external pressures.

It is the responsibility of those who realize how effectively massage can facilitate rehabilitation to see that patients receive this treatment. If it is not included in the physician's written prescription, often a tactful question will bring the value of massage to his attention.

Massage is a useful and integral part of the healing process. It should be used for psychological, physiological, mechanical, and reflex effects. Long before Christ, massage was used to relieve pain. A closer look at its history will help to clarify the development of massage.

Chapter 2

History of Massage

The art of massage was originated by the Chinese. Although the origin of Chinese medicine is lost in antiquity, it is assumed to have developed from folk medicine. It has many aspects in common with other Oriental traditions, such as Indian herbal medicine and Persian medicine.

In 1800 B.C. the Yoga cult in India used respiratory exercises for religious and healing purposes as recorded in the Veda books of wisdom. Egyptian, Persian, as well as Japanese medical literature is full of references to bath treatments of various kinds and massage. Hippocrates learned massage, as well as gymnastics, from his teacher Herodicus, the founder of medical gymnastics. Asclepiades, another eminent Greek physician, held the practice of this art in such esteem that he abandoned the use of all medicines, relying exclusively upon massage, which he claimed effects a cure by restoring to the nutritive fluids their natural, free movement. It was this physician who made the discovery that sleep might be induced by gentle stroking.

Plutarch tells us that Julius Caesar, a century before the Christian era, had himself daily pinched all over for neuralgia. It is well known that Julius Caesar was subject to a severe nervous disorder (epilepsy), and it is more than probable that his prodigious labors were only rendered possible by the aid derived from massage. Pliny, the great Roman naturalist, had himself rubbed for the relief of chronic asthma. Arrian recommended massage for horses and dogs, asserting that it would strengthen the limbs, render the hair soft and glossy, and cleanse the skin. After giving directions for massage of the legs, abdomen, and back, he directed that the treatment should be terminated in the following peculiar manner, indicating that he understood the value of nerve stretching, at least for dogs: "Lift her up by the tail, and give her a good stretching; let her go, and she will shake herself and show that she liked the treatment."

The ancient Greeks, Herodicus and Hippocrates, have left behind them prescriptions for massage and exercises. In 430 B.C. Hippocrates wrote, "It is necessary to rub the shoulder following reduction of a dislocated shoulder. It is necessary to rub the shoulder gently and smoothly." [1] The Greeks prescribed massage for their patients as well as for their athletes. They established elaborate bathhouses where exercises, massage, and baths were available, but these were patronized by the luxury loving to the exclusion of the health seekers. There is in the Pergamon Museum in Berlin a 2000-year-old alabaster relief from the palace of the Assyrian potentate, San Herib, which depicts a massage treatment as realistically as one seen in clinics today.

The pathfinders of ancient medicine were almost forgotten during the Middle Ages. Not until the sixteenth century was interest renewed when Ambroise Paré sought an anatomical and physiological foundation for mechanotherapy. From then on much was written about it, but nothing was actually done for mechanotherapy until the beginning of the last century, when medical gymnastics and massage took on a new life through the work of Per Henrik Ling of Sweden.

Ling was a fencing master and instructor of gymnastics. He began a study of massage after he had cured himself of rheumatism in the arm by percussions, and developed a method which consisted of massage and medical gymnastics without distinction between the two. It often combined both in a simultaneous application on the theory that massage is a form of passive gymnastics. He based his system on physiology, which was just then emerging as a science.

Through his ardent study and dedication, Ling won acceptance for his new ideas. His method became known as "The Ling System," or "The Swedish Movement Treatment." In 1813 the first college to include massage in the curriculum, called the Royal Gymnastic Central Institute, was established in Stockholm at the expense, and under the supervision, of the Swedish government. Ling died in 1839. His students subsequently published his theories, and, through them and the many foreign students at the Central Institute of Stockholm, Ling's system soon became known in a great part of the world.

Reputable institutes of massage and medical gymnastics sprang up in Germany, Austria, and France. People suffering from rheumatism

[1] Walter M. Solomon, "What is Happening to Massage," *Archives of Physical Medicine* (August 1950), pp. 521-23.

made yearly trips to the spas of Germany and France to take the "cure." This cure consisted of drinking gallons of mineral water, taking mineral baths, graduated exercise, and above all, massage. There was no place in America where one could get the same scientific attention. (This treatment is comparable to our present methods of salicylates, eliminating baths, graduated exercise, and massage.) It was a long time before the medical profession in England and America were willing to consider the matter seriously.

About 1880, Just Marie Marcellin Lucas-Championnière claimed that in fractures, the soft tissues as well as bony union should be considered from the start. Sir William Bennett of England was impressed with Lucas-Championnière's idea and started a revolutionary treatment with the use of massage at St. George's Hospital around 1899.

In 1900, Albert J. Hoffa published his book *Technik der Massage* in Germany. This book is still the most basic of all texts on massage, giving the clearest description of how to execute the stroke and advocating the procedures that underlie all modern techniques.[2]

The book by Max Bohm, *Massage, Its Principles and Techniques*, which was translated by Elizabeth Gould in 1913 also includes some interpretation of Hoffa's techniques.

In 1902, Dr. Douglas Graham, a strong advocate of massage, published *A Treatise on Massage, Its History, Mode of Application and Effects*. This text finally aroused the interest of the medical profession in the United States.

Sir Robert Jones, a leading orthopedic surgeon in England and president of the British Orthopedic Association, was an enthusiast for Lucas-Championnière's treatment of fractures. It was with his clinic at Southern Hospital in Liverpool that Mary McMillan was associated from 1911 to 1915. In the preface of his book James B. Mennell writes, "To Sir Robert Jones I am indebted for the valuable opportunity of working for him at the Special Military Surgical Hospital, Shepherd's Bush: and he has now added to his many kindnesses that of writing the Introduction which follows." [3] Thus the influence of Lucas-Championnière and Sir Robert Jones was exerted on both Miss McMillan and Dr. Mennell.

In 1917, Dr. E. G. Bracket and Dr. Joel Goldthwait were interested in the reconstruction work that was being done among the

[2] For the purposes of this study, Hoffa's book was translated for the author by Miss Ruth Friedlander.

[3] James B. Mennell, *Physical Treatment by Movement, Manipulation and Massage*, 5th ed. Philadelphia: The Blakiston Co., and London: J. A. Churchill, Ltd., 1945.

allied nations. They were the inaugurators of the Reconstruction Department of the United States Army in the early part of 1918. Short
intensive courses were arranged in order to train women to meet the
demand. McMillan served as chief aide at Walter Reed Army Hospital.
It was there that her influence on present techniques was of fundamental
importance.

McMillan received her special training in London at the National
Hospital for Nervous Diseases, at St. George's Hospital with Sir William
Bennett, and at St. Bartholomew's Hospital. After several years at the
Southern Hospital where she was in charge of massage and therapeutic
exercises at Greenbank Cripples' Home, she came to the United States
as director of Massage and Medical Gymnastics at Children's Hospital,
Portland, Maine. She then took over the responsibility of chief aide
at Walter Reed Hospital, and instructor of special war emergency
courses of Reed College Clinic for training reconstruction aides in
physiotherapy at Portland, Oregon. From 1921 to 1925, when her text
was written, she was director of physiotherapy (courses for graduates)
at Harvard Medical School.[4]

James B. Mennell wrote his text, *Physical Treatment by Movement, Manipulation and Massage*, in 1917 during World War I. It
has been revised several times; the fifth edition appeared in 1945. In
the first chapter of this text, he says,

> I have had opportunities of watching various workers—English,
> French, Swedish, Italian, Danish—and have tried to select all
> that I saw good, and to discard what seemed to me to be bad,
> in their methods.[5]

Mennell says in his introduction that he did not intend his book
to be seen as a text, but rather as what he considered the rationale of
massage treatment, and an endeavor to show the importance of care
and gentleness.

Mennell was a medical officer and lecturer of massage at the
Training School of St. Thomas's Hospital, London, England, from
1912 to 1935. Until his death in March, 1957, he worked constantly
to interest the medical field in the importance and usefulness of massage.

In 1929, Elisabeth Dicke developed an approach to massage
which emphasizes the use of specific reflex zones, a system known as
"Bindegewebsmassage." Her work will be discussed in detail in Chapter 17.

[4] Letter from Mary McMillan to Frances Tappan, June 19, 1948.

[5] Mennell, p. 2.

Beginning in 1937, Gertrude Beard contributed to the study of massage through her articles in the *Physical Therapy Review* and through her teaching at Northwestern University in Evanston, Illinois. Through the many graduates of this school who had the benefit of her teachings, her influence on massage techniques in America today has been profound. Although none of her writings are directly quoted in this text, many of her concepts have been included.

In 1944, Harold D. Storms published an article describing a massage stroke which he used both for diagnostic and therapeutic measures, particularly for fibrositic nodules. This technique (described in Chapter 10) is still widely used, especially in Canada and Puerto Rico.

James Cyriax defines a specific, limited approach to massage, recommending a type of friction that goes across the fibers of the structure being treated (Chapter 19). Because of his excellent illustrations and descriptions, many people in America today use this approach to massage.

Chapter 3

General Principles of Massage

These general principles are derived from the author's experience as well as research of the literature of other massage techniques.

A number of basic principles should be kept in mind at all times. First, the operator should have knowledge of the patient's complete diagnosis, so that massage functions not as an isolated method, but as part of the patient's total treatment plan. Second, physical contact establishes a close relationship between operator and patient. This contact should be understanding and sympathetic, but never personal.

PERSONAL APPEARANCE

Personal appearance of the operator should be above reproach. Clothing should be neat, clean, and comfortable, allowing freedom of motion.

CARE OF HANDS

The hands are all important in giving a massage. They should be washed before every treatment. Rings should not be worn since they might scratch the patient. The fingernails should be cut so short that one cannot see them if the hands are held up with the palm toward the face.

The hands should always be warm and dry before they touch the patient. If necessary, they can be warmed beneath an infrared lamp for a few moments or dried by applying powder to them. They can also be warmed by hot water or by rubbing them briskly together before touching the patient.

POSTURE

Good posture of the operator will avoid fatigue and backache. The weight should rest evenly on both feet with the body in good postural alignment. When massaging a large area, the weight should shift from one foot to the other. A good operator can apply pressure by a shift of body weight instead of using muscle strength.

TREATMENT TABLE

The treatment table should be the right height to allow for correct postural balance of weight. In addition, a set of platforms ranging from two to six inches in height can be very useful. These platforms should be of adequate width and length to allow for the complete stance of the operator, who can place his or her hands on the part to be treated without leaning over or reaching up.

The treatment table should be of wood or metal with a firm pad or mattress, but without springs. Even in the patient's home, one ideally should seek a firm surface, such as a tabletop, and not treat the patient in a bed which offers no firm support. There are, of course, numerous exceptions to this ideal. A nurse, for example, often gives a back massage to a bedridden patient.

POSITIONING THE PATIENT

Specific positioning will be discussed with each unit; however, there are certain general precautions which should be considered. *Solid support must be given, extending distally and proximally as far as the joints on either side of the injury.*

It cannot be too greatly emphasized that the position should always be one that is comfortable for the patient. There are certain stretching positions that make use of the effect of gravity to put a slight stretch on individual muscles which might need it, but even these should not be so uncomfortable that the patient cannot relax.

In general, the part to be massaged should be elevated in order to allow gravity to assist the mechanical effects of the treatment and make the increased venous return that much easier. Exceptions to this rule will be mentioned later.

At no time should the patient have to exert muscular effort to hold the part being treated in position or to hold the draping about himself. Sometimes sandbags or rolled towels may be used to brace the limb.

DRAPING

Tight clothing should be removed and a sheet or towel used to cover the parts of the body not being treated. In arranging the draping the patient should not be unnecessarily exposed to the point where it may cause embarrassment. He or she should be at ease to enjoy the treatment and feel confidence in the person who is about to administer this treatment.

Movements should be businesslike and the operator should assure the patient that he is capable and has a professional interest in the problems of the patient. The operator, of course, should never lean on the patient while reaching across the table to arrange the draping.

If the patient is unable to relax because of positioning, lack of adequate support to the part, apprehension concerning the treatment, tight or uncomfortable draping, or discomfort due to being too warm or too cold, the desirable effects of the massage may not be accomplished. Specific positions and basic supportive measures will be discussed later when the massage of each area of the body is described.

LUBRICANTS

The purpose of a lubricant is to avoid uncomfortable friction between the hand of the operator and the skin of the patient. Older texts may suggest shaving the part to be massaged if superfluous hair interferes with the treatment, but such procedure is no longer recommended.

There are many types of lubricants. Any lanolin-base cold cream may be used because of its nonirritating qualities. Mineral oil or baby oil may be used, according to preference. Any of the creams or oils can be cleaned from the patient with alcohol. If the primary effect of the massage has been to obtain relaxation, soap and warm water can be used instead of alcohol to remove the lubricant. Care should be taken not to stain the patient's clothes by leaving lubricants on the skin.

With dry skin it is often best *not* to remove the lubricant. In such instances the patient can be advised to wear clothing that can be stained without concern.

When massaging stump ends, 70 percent alcohol is often used. In these cases stimulation and toughening of the stump is desired.

Some patients may be allergic to a lubricant. This can usually be eliminated by changing the type of lubricant. Persistent rash should, of course, be called to the attention of a doctor.

Cocoa butter is often used on scar tissue caused by burns or where skin nutrition is indicated, but it has a higher melting point and is, therefore, more inconvenient to use. Olive oil may also be used for skin nutrition, but it becomes rancid quickly and is difficult to keep for general use.

Powder is very useful because it is not so difficult to cleanse following the treatment. An odorless powder should be used.

Some people prefer to massage with no lubricant, but if this method is used, care must be taken to be sure that the superficial hair of the skin is not pulled and that the hands of the person giving the massage are not moist.

Strong commercial ointments for "rubbing" often produce blisters if used in conjunction with heat and are more irritating to skin that has been made sensitive by serious illness or injury. Therefore, the use of such ointments is not encouraged. If such stronger ointments have been used by the patient before coming for treatment, care must be taken to wash them off prior to administering any heat or massage.

Too much lubricant prevents firm contact, and the hands will only slip over the surface of the skin. It is better to have too little than too much. It remains a common error to use lubricants too generously. Many authorities advocate massage without any at all. This author advocates its proper usage and recommends some practice without the use of lubricant.

In the early phase of learning massage, tension often causes nervous perspiration of the hands. A solution of alum and alcohol will reduce the amount of moisture and lessen the need for powder.

PRESSURE AND RHYTHM

Pressure should be adjusted to the contours of the body and care used over bony areas. All strokes should be rhythmical. The pressure strokes should end with a swing off in a small half circle so that the rhythm will not be broken by an abrupt stop.

Consider the patient's threshold of pain or discomfort. All massage should begin lightly, even in patients who have little involvement or in athletic situations where the person being treated is absolutely normal. As the depth of the stroke increases, the operator should watch the patient carefully to be sure that pressure is not greater than can be tolerated.

If a muscle tightens under the touch, it has probably been given too severe treatment or so light a touch that it "tickles."

It is important to maintain contact with the patient once the treatment begins. The hands should not break contact with the skin in deep stroking and kneading except on changing areas. Even though some strokes require an actual loss of contact, the rhythm of the loss should infer that the treatment is a continuing process. Mennell mentions in his description of superficial stroking that the stroke through the air should take the same length of time as the stroke on the body.[1]

Treatment should not be interrupted. To stop suddenly to adjust the draping, to dry the hands because they have too much lubricant on them, or to turn and talk to someone is upsetting to the patient and to the rhythmical procedure. The telephone should be answered by someone else, unless emergencies arise. Even then, the stop should not be sudden. Do not lift the hands in the middle of an effleurage stroke. Cover the patient to keep him or her warm during the interruption.

Stopping the treatment in order to move around the table or bed to treat the other side should not be done unless both legs or arms are being treated. Neither should one ask the patient to change position once the treatment has begun. One must learn how to approach the patient from almost any angle, since many involvements make it difficult or impossible for the patient to move about easily.

Follow the Venous Flow

The pressure strokes should be in line with the venous flow, followed by a return stroke without pressure.

DURATION

Treatment time is an individual decision. Contrary to older texts stating a routine or set time, modern operators now follow the advice of Mennell and adjust the time to the needs of each patient.

REST

Rest for the patient following treatment is always advised, especially in cases where the involved part is a weight-bearing limb which must be put to work as soon as the patient is ambulatory.

Length of time for this rest must be judged by the operator. If

[1] Mennell, p. 34.

there is swelling in a dependent limb, the resting time should be long enough to permit reduction of swelling before ambulation is attempted.

SUMMARY

One should avoid treating patients without complete knowledge of the diagnosis. Personal appearance should be above reproach; hands should be warm and clean; good postural alignment is necessary. The patient should be comfortable and warm, and in a position which is functional for the operator. All tight clothing should be removed and draping should protect the modesty of the patient. Lubricants may at times be convenient but are never absolutely necessary.

Chapter 4

Effects of Massage

Massage is a healing art. It is a unique way of communicating without words. Through touching another person, we may communicate the fact that we *care*; we empathize with him; we want to share our energy with him.

Dolores Krieger, Ph.D., R.N., in 1972 proved in a controlled study that hemoglobin could be increased through the use of Therapeutic Touch.[1] Dr. Krieger writes that:

> We can help each other and we can help ourselves through Therapeutic Touch. Whether through the channeling of natural energy sources on the physical level, or the recruiting of human energy sources on the psychodynamic level, the message is clear: a new age is dawning in which we can intelligently cooperate with nature, in which we can intelligently cooperate with each other.[2]

In suggesting as an underlying drive the concept of a need to help, Dr. Krieger further states:

> A need to help wells up from the same psychodynamic depths from which arose the stimuli that guided early man not merely to mate, but to form the nuclear family in which attributes of love and caring and protection from harm were nurtured. This need to help is probably the most humane of human characteristics. It lies very close to the central motivations that bring most people into health care.

Krieger's research is concerned with Therapeutic Touch, which derives, but is not the same as, the laying-on of hands. She says it is the

[1] Dolores Krieger, "The Relationship of Touch with Intent to Help or to Heal, Ss In-vivo Hemoglobin Values: A Study in Personalized Interactions," *Proc. American Nurses Assn., 9th Nursing Research Conference.* Kansas City: The Assoc., 1973.

[2] Dolores Krieger, "Nursing Research for a New Age," *Nursing Times,* April 1976, pp. 1-7.

uniquely human act of *concern* of one individual for another which is characterized by touching in an act that incorporates an intent to help or to heal the person so touched.

> To be truly therapeutic, this act must be deeply motivated in the best interests of the person who is being touched. The person doing the touching must be educable, for although the act seems quite simple, it is in fact quite complex and the toucher must be able to understand the underlying dynamics of these complexities. One must, for instance, be able to learn to recognize certain cues to subtle levels of consciousness in order to be intelligently aware of the processes, conscious and unconscious, which may be set in motion; and one must be able to develop the insight to recognize whether this mode of therapeutics is meeting the patient's needs or buttressing one's own ego structure. Therapeutic Touch is a tool frequently used by those who deliver health care, either knowledgeably or unconsciously. Since we are responsible for our acts, therefore, it behooves us to understand the basis for this particular mode of therapeutics as well as we would understand the underlying dynamics of any pharmaceuticals that might be given, or any other procedure in which we might engage ourselves.

Since massage is most certainly "touching," Krieger's ideas concerning the importance of the way touching is done to promote healing have a direct relationship to the touching involved in massage as one of the healing procedures.

The effects of massage are not only psychological but also mechanical, physiological, and reflexive in nature. By massage, stimulation is provided to the exteroceptors of the skin and proprioceptive receptors of the underlying tissues. Relief of pain is brought about through any one of these effects, or by a combination of any of them.

MECHANICAL EFFECTS OF MASSAGE

Mechanically, massage assists the venous flow of blood, encourages lymphatic flow, reduces certain types of edema, provides gentle stretching of tissue, and relieves subcutaneous scar tissue.

Assists Venous Flow

Normally the constant contraction of muscles as people move about pushes against the veins, pressing the blood on toward the heart.

When this normal activity is inhibited by injury or illness, the resulting decreased circulation adds another complication to the already disturbed metabolism of the tissues involved.

The mechanical effect of deep stroking on the superficial veins in the direction of the venous flow is easily observed in many persons. The resulting decreased venous pressure provides a favorable situation for increased arterial circulation. When capillary pressure is reduced, the potential for filtration into the extracellular spaces is decreased; thus the load on the lymphatics is also decreased and the possibility of fibrosis is diminished.

When possible, gravity should be considered to assist, rather than inhibit, the flow of blood within the veins. The valves within the veins prevent any backflow of blood once it has been encouraged forward. This direct mechanical effect includes mainly the more superficial veins.

Assists Lymphatic Flow

Lymph is a viscid fluid that moves slowly through the lymphatic system. The lymphatics are, for the most part, noncontractile. Movement of lymph depends upon outside forces such as the contraction of muscles and pressure generated by filtration of fluid from the capillaries. Immobility due to pain or paralysis seriously interferes with lymph drainage. The lymphatics have a lower pressure and slower flow than the venous flow.

Massage can encourage lymphatic flow, preventing the edema that often occurs with inactivity. Since lymph is viscid and moves slowly, massage strokes should be slow and rhythmical when used for this purpose. Massage is an excellent mechanical substitute when normal muscular functioning has been interrupted, but active exercise should be encouraged as soon as possible. According to Ladd, Kottke, and Blanchard, massage will increase lymphatic flow, but active exercise will do this more efficiently.[3]

Stretches

Another mechanical effect of massage is the stretching of superficial tissues. When combined with a passive-exercise type of stretching it will encourage the patient to relax and allow further passive stretching of a muscle that has become shortened.

[3] M. P. Ladd, F. J. Kottke, and R. S. Blanchard, "Studies of the Effect of Massage on the Flow of Lymph From the Foreleg of the Dog," *Arch. Phys. Med.* 33: 10 (Oct. 1952), pp. 604-12.

Loosens Scar Tissue

Subcutaneous scar tissue can at times be loosened by careful and persistent friction. Once it has formed, deeper scarring in connective tissue *cannot* be relieved by massage. Massage can prevent scarring *to some degree* by not allowing stagnation of tissue edema following injury, thus preventing fibrosis.

Total Blood Flow

Massage does not increase total blood flow nor influence total body metabolism unless it is too traumatic to be tolerated by an individual with an abnormality. After very deep stroking there is some increase in blood flow of the massaged extremity but no change in the contralateral extremity.

Obesity

The old idea that obesity can be reduced by massage has been dispelled. Massage too traumatic for humans to tolerate might bruise the adipose tissue, necessitating replacement with new tissue. However, this new tissue would only be *more* adipose tissue. As a "come on" in reducing salons, massage is combined with steam baths which reduce the water content of the body through excessive perspiration, thus showing an immediate loss of weight on the salon scale. Massage can only induce a psychological feeling of well-being for such customers.

Muscle-mass, Strength, and Motion

Massage is ineffective in delaying loss of mass and strength following nerve injuries. It will not hasten the recovery of sensation, nor will it produce a better histologic picture. It will, however, accelerate voluntary and reflex action once the nerve injury has begun to recover and reenervation is present. In such cases massage should be combined with passive and active reeducational exercise.

Therefore, massage is a part of the patient's total rehabilitation program, not an independent treatment to be used by itself. Any evaluation of the usefulness of massage must consider its role in total patient care.

PHYSIOLOGICAL EFFECTS

The student of massage should have some understanding of the physiology of the heart and circulation, particularly the peripheral circulation and the return flow of blood and lymph, as taught in basic physiology courses.

The purpose of this discussion is to summarize and review basic physiology which relates to massage.

Metabolism

Metabolically, the muscles maintain a chemical balance through normal activity. As they contract they rid themselves of toxic products by "milking" these acids into the lymphatic and venous flow. As they contract they assist this lymphatic and venous flow toward the heart through mechanical pressure which pushes blood and lymph through channels where valves prevent a backflow. Thus these by-products are carried away.

As the muscles relax, fresh blood flows into them, bringing necessary nutrition to the area.

Overactivity disturbs this balance by not allowing sufficient relaxation time for the inflow of nutritive products. At the same time, due to exertion, toxic products are formed faster than they can be eliminated. Thus the muscle is loaded with irritant acids.

Underactivity also disturbs this balance by not providing the "milking" effect to assist the venous and lymphatic return. Thus the irritant products which form within the muscles are not carried away as they should be and the muscle becomes more or less "stagnant."

Following extreme activity, these irritant acids can be hastened back into the venous return by massage. Often the "lameness" that follows abnormal activity could be lessened or prevented by massage immediately following the activity, since the muscles themselves are inhibited by fatigue.

In many situations, where partial or total muscular inactivity occurs, massage can mechanically assist the "milking" process. However, it can never replace normal muscular activity.

Venostasis

Muscular inactivity can bring about a venostasis, particularly in the dependent limbs where gravity inhibits the normal venous return. Other causes for venostasis may be varicosity, thrombosis, or pressure on the vessels by edema within the surrounding tissues (due to local inflammation or due to the venostasis itself).

It is obvious that massage should *not* be given if there is a possibility of spreading inflammation, if there is a possibility of dislodging a thrombus, thus causing embolism, or if there is such obstruction that the mechanical assistance of massage could not improve the venous flow. Massage given *first* to the proximal aspects of an injured limb will insure that these circulatory pathways are open enough to carry the venous flow along toward the heart.

Edema

Several causes for edema can be found in *The Living Body* by Best and Taylor. The following is quoted directly from this excellent physiology text:

> An increase in the quantity of tissue fluid to the point where it causes a readily detectable increase in volume of a part is called *edema*. It is most frequently seen in the skin and subcutaneous tissues, as a symptom of heart or of kidney disease. When the edema is well marked, the skin appears "puffy" and, when one presses it with a finger, a dent or pit is left which takes a little time to level up again.
>
> Edema is due to an imbalance of those factors regulating the interchange of fluids between the vessels and the tissue spaces. . . . It may result, therefore, from any of the following causes, (a) increased capillary pressure, as in heart disease, (b) reduced plasma osmotic pressure, as in chronic kidney disease, (c) increased permeability of the capillary wall as in acute kidney disease or as a result of certain poisons, e.g. histamine, (d) obstruction of the lymph channels (lymphatic edema).[4]

These types of edema should *not* be treated with massage, unless in a specific instance a physician gives careful instructions for an unusual situation.

There are, however, certain types of edema where massage can be of some assistance. Already mentioned is the venostasis caused by muscular inactivity, which may be due to paralysis, injury, or illness. If there is no actual obstruction (such as thrombus) and the edema is caused only by the inactivity of the part, there can be no harm in massaging edema from the foot and ankle. An example is a well-healed fracture of the femur which is not yet weight-bearing and the leg is allowed to hang down in a dependent position with little or no muscular activity. Without adequate instruction for nonweight-bearing exercises and advice for part-time elevation of the leg (so that gravity can assist the venous return), massage alone will be of little assistance. Massage is not in itself a total treatment, but contributes an important part to the total treatment.

[4] From *The Living Body*, Fourth Edition, by Charles Herbert Best and Norman Burke Taylor. Reprinted by permission of Holt, Rinehart and Winston, Inc., Copyright 1958, pp. 101-2.

In cases of recent injury, where edema is evident due to torn tissues and internal bleeding, massage to the injured area would only encourage further bleeding and more swelling. If massage is indicated at all, it should be given only to areas proximal to the injury, or given so superficially that no further injury would be caused. Massage to any area exhibiting this type of edema should *never* be given unless ordered by a physician, who will indicate when sufficient healing has taken place to tolerate such treatment.

REFLEX EFFECTS

Recently an active interest has developed in the reflex effects of massage. Sir James MacKenzie defines the reflex process as, "that vital process which is concerned in the reception of a stimulus by one organ or tissue and its conduction to another organ, which on receiving a stimulus produces the effect."[5] In massage the hands stimulate the sensory receptors of the skin and subcutaneous tissues, causing reflex effects. The stimuli pass along the afferent fibers of the peripheral nervous system to the spinal cord; from there, it is conceivable that these stimuli may disperse through the central and autonomic nervous systems, producing various effects in any zone supplied from the same segment of the spinal cord. Some of these effects are capillary vasodilatation or constriction, relaxation or stimulation of voluntary muscle contraction, and gooseflesh. In addition, there is the possible sedation or stimulation of sensory reception with sedation or stimulation of pain. In extreme cases reflex effects may be severe. They could cause nausea, vomiting, and depression of the heart's action with resulting pallor and sweating.

On this principle Elisabeth Dicke organized the specific routine described in her text, *Meine Bindegewebsmassage*. If these viscerocutaneous effects are possible it can be seen that beneficial effects from massage of specific zones could be produced with controlled results.

Mirriam Jacobs discussed the reflex effects of massage as follows:[6]

The increased circulation by way of improved superficial venous and lymphatic flow is an effect of deep pressure produced by stroking or compression movements. Mechanical pressure

[5] J. MacKenzie, *Angina Pectoris* (London: Henry Frowde and Hodder and Stoughton, 1923), p. 47.

[6] Miriam Jacobs, "Massage for the Relief of Pain: Anatomical and Physiological Considerations," *Phys. Therapy Rev.*, 40: 2 (Feb. 1960), pp. 96-97. Reprinted with the kind permission of Miriam Jacobs and the *Physical Therapy Review*.

from stroking movements probably also produces direct effects upon the capillaries resulting in capillary contraction as seen in the "white" reaction following mechanical stimulation of the skin. It is said to be of capillary origin and is not dependent upon nerves. According to the standard physiology texts, it may be a direct response of the capillaries to irritation or to some substance liberated as a result of the mechanical stimulus. With firmer pressure, a "red" reaction appears. This is the result of capillary dilation and is not dependent upon nervous mechanisms. Stronger stimuli or repeated stimuli produce a "red flare" and is due to dilation of the arteriole. It is thought that dilation of the arteriole may be due to a local axon reflex mechanism (1). With an intense stimulus (which is not considered a desirable massage procedure in this country) a wheal may be formed. This "triple response" red reaction, red flare and wheal formation is believed to be brought about by a diffusion of a substance liberated by the cells of the skin in response to mechanical stimulation. The substance bears a resemblance to histamine in its effects; capillary dilation by its direct effects, arteriole dilation by the axon reflex, and finally a wheal due to the increased capillary permeability and the release of fluid.

The existence of vasoconstrictor nerve fibers which increase the tone of the arterioles is unquestioned. Their cells of origin are located in the intermediolateral column of gray matter of the thoracic and upper lumbar cord and their fibers pass via the anterior roots to synapse in the chain ganglia via the white rami; they rejoin the segmental spinal nerves via the gray rami to be distributed to the vessels of the skin and muscles. The anatomy of the vasodilator fibers is confusing and debatable. The vasoconstrictor fibers are limited for the most part to the sympathetic system; the vasodilator fibers may not be restricted to the parasympathetic system as is often described. Barron suggests that vasodilator fibers are distributed not only via the parasympathetic outflow but they are also found co-mingled with the vasoconstrictor fibers of the sympathetic outflow (2). Another group of vasodilator fibers are said to be intermingled with the afferents of the spinal nerves. At the periphery, an afferent fiber from a receptor in the skin may give off a collateral to the arterioles of the vascular bed of the skin. Thus, local stimulation of the skin sets up (in addition to the afferent impulses to the central nervous system) an axon reflex that acts upon the arterioles. That vasodilation does follow experimentally produced antidromic stimulation (causing impulses to flow back to the receptor) of the dorsal root is generally accepted. The question that is debated is whether impulses are normally set up in the central ends of the dorsal root afferents, for neural control of the blood vessels of the skin. Such an antidromic effect could explain the effects of massage;

i.e., peripheral stimulation of the sensory afferents resulting in reflex dilation of the arterioles of the muscles and vascular bed of the skin.

Bayliss has shown that stimulation of the sensory afferent nerves from the limbs in animals brings about vasodilation due to inhibition of the local vasoconstrictors as well as excitation of the local vasodilators, an effect comparable to reciprocal innervation seen in skeletal muscle (2). Thus the blood supply increased by the sensory stimulation of massage may be a combination of excitation of the vasodilators and inhibition of the vasoconstrictors.

Barron suggests that evidence is also accumulating which indicates that there are pressure sensitive fibers intermingled in other nerves of the blood vessels of the skin and viscera which if activated bring about a fall in blood pressure through vasodilatation of the splanchnic region (2). He further states that stimulation of the sciatic or other mixed nerves by cooling, activation by weak stimuli or mechanical stimuli may cause vasodilation of the splanchnic area (2). This might explain some of the visceral effects claimed by the advocates of Bindegewebsmassage which may be termed a weak stimulus (3).

Deep pain following ischemia resulting from sustained muscle contraction may be relieved by massage through the improved circulation afforded by, 1) the mechnical pressure on superficial venous and lymphatic channels, and 2) reflex dilatation through stimulation of the cutaneous afferents mediating touch and pressure. Another possibility for the relief of pain may be mediated through another mechanism. The stretch or tension, placed on the tendons and fascia surrounding the muscles during the stretching and compression movements, as in petrissage, may have an inhibitory effect on sustained muscle contraction. It is a well known fact that a "cramped muscle" can be relaxed by stretching it or by deep kneading. Impulses from the tendon sensory organs (probably Golgi tendon organs) and perhaps also from the fascia and adjacent joint structures, which are activated by stretch, produce powerful central inhibition of the neurons controlling that muscle. This effect has been called the inverse myotatic reflex (4). Relaxation and the relief of pain of sustained muscle contraction by massage and traction might possibly be explained on this basis.

References for Miss Jacobs' Article

1. Bard, Philip, *Medical Physiology*. C. V. Mosby Co., St. Louis, 1956, pp. 158–59.

2. Barron D. J., "Physiology of the Organs of Circulation of the Blood and Lymph." Sec. VI in *Textbook of Physi-*

ology, edited by J. F. Fulton. W. B. Saunders Co., Philadelphia, 1955, pp. 566–87, 755–94.

3.   Ebner M., "Peripheral circulatory disturbances: treatment by massage of connective tissues in reflex zones," *Brit. J. Phys. Med.*, Vol. 19, August, 1956, pp. 176–80.

4.   Lloyd, D. P. C., "Principles of Nervous Activity." Sec. I in *Textbook of Physiology*, edited by J. E. Fulton. W. B. Saunders Co., 1955, pp. 104–9.

EFFECTS OF MASSAGE ON THE SKIN

Since the hands contact the skin when massage is done, the effects of this treatment on the skin should be considered. One of the major effects is the contact this pressure makes with the sensory nerve endings. Usually massage is sedative and these effects are therefore beneficial. If, however, there is a nerve injury present which makes these sensory nerve endings extremely hypersensitive, so sensitive in fact that massage does not bring sedation but only increases the pain of the patient, it is then contraindicated. It would not be given unless the operator could lower the pain threshold of the patient by an extremely technical approach. Occasionally these patients can tolerate a firm contact better than a superficial one, and if such were the case, continued massage might be indicated.

The condition of the skin following extreme injury is often abnormal. Parts which have been in a cast will have layers of dead skin under which tender, new skin has developed. In cases where the skin has been burned, massage would not be indicated until adequate scar tissue has formed. Decision as to when this type of tissue (and it may be a skin graft) may be treated is made by the physician in charge.

Because the skin helps remove excretory products its pores must be kept open. The friction of massage will create heat which invites perspiration and increases sebaceous excretions. The skin also carries out a certain amount of respiration (exchanging carbon dioxide and oxygen) and can be assisted by massage after the part has been in a cast and the normal function of the skin has been inhibited. Massage in these cases helps the skin return to normal function.

If there are layers of dead skin inhibiting the normal functions of skin, they can best be removed by first subjecting the part to whirlpool, followed by massage.

Occasionally a patient's skin will react to massage by breaking out or showing infections of the hair follicles. In the presence of such infections, massage is discontinued until reordered by the physician, or the type of lubricant is changed, or occasionally massage with no lubricant at all is given.

Summary

Massage increases venous and lymphatic flow; reduces certain types of edema; provides stretching of tissue; relieves subcutaneous scar tissue; improves nutrition through the skin by the application of special lubricants; increases perspiration, thus removing excretory products; helps to remove dry scaly skin following casting; and assists soft tissue toward normal metabolic balance. In addition, there are reflex effects from the stimulation of sensory receptors of the skin and subcutaneous tissues.

Chapter 5

Creating Positive Attitudes Toward Healing

The art of healing is a two-way street. Massage given by one who includes the patient as a partner will be remarkably more effective than one given as a mere technique of body manipulation. One who devotes total attention by communicating concern, empathy, and sincere desire to promote the healing process will spur a patient to participate in the effort toward regaining good health.

The mutual aim is to replace patient dependency with collaborative effort by patient and operator. To establish this relationship, the patient must participate in discussions which include exchange of ideas, rather than simply receive instructions given by the operator. Such an approach will strengthen positive attitudes and exclude feelings of despair.

A pleasant atmosphere, the exchange of laughter, a sense of strength or determination, and feelings of love will strongly encourage the human body toward its own constant search for homeostasis. The body itself will then produce more complicated and comprehensive chemotherapy than is available at any medical center in the world, be it via Eastern or Western medical approaches (see Endorphins, Chapter 6).

While giving massage one can encourage the patient to understand the potential source of healing in his own consciousness. He can be encouraged not to be helpless, passive, depressed, or desperate, but rather capable and active in his own treatment. Skillful encouragement can stimulate the human body's own defense and healing mechanisms.

Current research done with plants, animals, and human beings is proving that positive effects are possible through the "laying-on of hands." "Lay thy hand upon it" goes as far back as Sushruta Samhita.[1] In an experiment conducted in 1964, Bernard Grad used barley seeds that had been soaked in saline to stimulate a "sick" condition.[2] Oskar Estebany worked with Grad as a "healer" and held flasks of water as he would were he doing laying-on of hands. An identical saline flask of barley seeds was not treated by the laying-on of hands. The seeds held by Estebany sprouted more quickly, grew taller, and contained more chlorophyll. (Grad reported p. .001.)

In the book *The Secret Life of Plants*,[3] Peter Tompkins and Christopher Bird record how Cleve Backster proved without doubt that plants respond if touched with affection. By using lie detector equipment he confirmed Grad's studies that plants respond to loving care and soft music in a positive way. Conversely, they respond negatively to hard rock music and feelings of hate.

In Eastern cultures the transference of attitudes between the healer and subject is believed to occur via a state of matter for which the Western culture has neither a word nor a concept. It is called *prana* in Sanskrit. The nearest translation in the West is "vitality" or "vigor." The Chinese called it *Chi*, which translates into "energy." Regardless of what it is called, however, this phenomenon refers to the balanced functioning of the human body and the vital life force of energy, which keeps people in good physiological and psychological health. Advocates of this concept believe the healer can transfer his own positive energy to the patient through touch (via any medical approach—pulse reading, acupuncture or more modern medical methods) to return the patient to normal health. They also believe that it is absolutely necessary for the patient to have faith in the healer and to possess a strong will to get well.

Krieger's recent controlled study proved that therapeutic touch or again, the laying-on of hands, is a uniquely effective human act. Her results showed significant measurable changes in hemoglobin values.[4] By touching with the intent to help or heal, the patient would feel heat

---

[1] Greed Mayno, *The Healing Hand*. Cambridge, Mass.: Harvard University Press, 1975.

[2] Bernard Grad, et al. "A Telekenetic Effect on Plant Growth, Part 2. Experiments Involving Treatment with Saline in Stoppered Bottles," *Int. Journal of Parapsychol.* 6:473-98, 1964.

[3] Peter Tompkins and Christopher Bird, *The Secret Life of Plants*. New York: Avon, 1973, p. 19.

[4] Dolores Krieger, "Nursing Research for a New Age," *Nursing Times*, April 1976, pp. 1-7.

within the area beneath the hand. Patients reported feeling profoundly relaxed and having a sense of well-being.

In "Anatomy of an Illness," Norman Cousins records how he became, with his doctor, William Hitzig, a participant in the accomplishment of his own recovery. Together they proved that a cheerful atmosphere and an open-minded exchange of ideas related to recovery actually reduced the high sedimentation rate causing his illness. He achieved an almost complete recovery and returned to functional health.[5]

Such attitudes do not develop without concentrated effort on the part of the healer and the one desiring to be healed. All patients are individuals with problems, physical problems that create mental attitudes that may vary all the way from complete rejection of treatment to complete cooperation. Before treating a patient, explain what his treatment will accomplish. Always try to find out what the patient is thinking and feeling by listening more than talking. Work *with* the patient rather than saying, "Now *I* want you to . . . ." Inspire the patient's confidence with a positive attitude that implies that your knowledge and skill are available for him to receive. This also means that the healer cannot afford to display any negative feelings of his own regardless of anger or rudeness on the part of the patient. A healer's firm, controlled strength of character can guide the patient toward acceptance and belief that the treatment is for his benefit.

John Newbern is credited with the adage that people can be divided into three groups: "Those who make things happen, those who watch things happen, and those who wonder what happened!" [6] It is the operator's responsibility to encourage the patient to do all in his power to "make things happen."

Summary

It should be firmly emphasized that the terms "healing" or "the healer" do not refer to the mystical or occult. It is a well-known fact that one is much more likely to achieve the balance of health and happiness with positive attitudes than with negative feelings. The importance of touch, particularly as it relates to massage, can make the difference between healing and the lack of it.

[5] Norman Cousins, "Anatomy of an Illness (as Perceived by the Patient)," *Saturday Review,* May 28, 1977, pp. 4-6, 48-51.

[6] See Krieger, pp. 1-7.

Chapter 6

Results of Recent Research

ENDORPHINS

The physiology of pain and how to relieve it has led to the discovery of endorphin (*endo*genous *morphine*). The discovery of endorphins grew out of identification of opiate receptors in the brain and other tissues.[1] That is, sites on the cell surface specifically combine with the opiates in order to produce their characteristic biological effects of analgesia and euphoria.

Structurally related peptides present in the brain, pituitary, or both, and a low molecular weight peptide in blood, mimic some actions of opiates.[2] Pertinent evidence is now starting to accumulate in two areas. Not only are emotions related to the flow of neurotransmitters in the brain, thus directly affecting the transmission of pain signals, but the brain itself is capable of producing a powerful analgesic substance. This substance, endorphin, is five to 10 times more powerful than morphine and has recently been shown to inhibit the transmission of pain signals through the spinal cord. Although evidence is still scanty, it seems likely that many pain-killing techniques have this common denominator, the ability to stimulate endorphin.[3]

[1] Jean L. Marx, "Neurobiology: Researchers High on Endogenous Opiates," *Science*, September 24, 1976, p. 1227.

[2] *Ibid.*

[3] Julie Wang, "Breaking Out of the Pain Trap," *Psychology Today*, July 1977, p. 79.

Dr. Avram Goldstein, professor of pharmacology at Stanford University and director of the Addiction Research Foundation, Palo Alto, California, is a leading researcher in opioid peptides (endorphins) in the pituitary and brain.[4]

His investigation has been directed toward characterizing the pituitary opioid peptides that behave as typical opioid agonists. Naloxone is a synthetic drug that is a specific antagonist of endorphins and blocks their effect. Laboratory animals given naloxone feel more intense pain than others not receiving the drug. Goldstein found peptides of different molecular size could display opioid activity.

Goldstein also says, "The brain is basically a chemical organ. Those many thousands of millions of brain cells talk to each other in chemical language." He calls endorphins, "the morphine within." [5]

Enkephalins are specific pentopeptides belonging to the endorphin class. Researchers think that enkephalins may be true neurotransmitters. Enkephalins and the larger endorphins and possibly some as yet unidentified substance, may be concentrated in discrete regions of the brain, some of which are associated with pain perception, or of the generation of moods.[6]

Snyder, with Candace Pert and Michael Kuhar, used a radio autographic technique to show nonrandom-type distribution of receptors. Snyder and Pert also found that the receptors are located in the subcellular fraction of brain cells that contains the synaptic membranes. This synapse is the logical site for receptors for neurotransmitters. Distribution of enkephalins parallels that of the receptors.[7]

Endorphins have also been shown to have an effect on mood in experiments by Goldstein at the Addiction Research Center.[8] Normal people were put in stressful, anxiety-producing situations. Some were given naloxone, which blocks endorphins, while others were given a placebo. Those receiving the placebo experienced a relaxation response once the stressful situation ended; those given naloxone remained keyed-up and anxious. This seems to demonstrate the tranquilizing effect of endorphin. Goldstein says, "Maybe we all carry our own dope around in our heads."

[4] Avram Goldstein, "Opioid Peptides (Endorphins) in Pituitary and Brain," *Science*, 193 (September 17, 1976), p. 1081.

[5] Stanford University Medical Center, "The Morphine Within," *The Healing Arts*, 7:1 (1977), p. 7.

[6] Marx, p. 1228.

[7] *Ibid.*

[8] "The Morphine Within," p. 8.

Research into enkephalins may also be a major breakthrough in bridging the gap between *acupuncture* and *neurophysiology*. The Chinese have used acupuncture for mood elevation for thousands of years, long before anyone knew about endorphins. Acupuncture (peripheral stimulation of the loci) produces analgesia. For example, accurate stimulation of the ear point, or "Lung," relieves the symptoms of drug withdrawal in animals and man, between 10 and 30 minutes after onset of stimulation. This time lag indicates that acupuncture mechanisms involve the production and release of endogenous humeral factors.[9]

Research has been done with the transfusion of whole blood, serum, and cerebrospinal fluid in rabbits, rats and dogs who had been given a specific acupuncture stimulation. Rabbits were given acupuncture and then bled, with their serum transfused to other rabbits. Analgesia developed in 70 percent of the recipients in the same limb as that of the donor. This left 30 percent who did not respond. Serum from nonacupunctured rabbits had no effect when transfused to other rabbits.[10]

There is still another peptide (anodynin) which produces analgesia that lasts longer than enkephalins. Removal of the pituitary glands of rats results in almost complete disappearance of anodynin from blood. Researchers believe it may be involved in the activity of opiate receptors in nerves of peripheral tissues, and are studying the effects of stress, pain, sleep, and other physiological states on the concentration of anodynin in the blood. Anodynin may be released into the bloodstream with acupuncture.

Julie Wang, in "Breaking Out of the Pain Trap," [11] refers to other ways that acupuncture might be effective. Studies show that dietary and chemical depletion of brain serotonin levels increases sensitivity to pain. Both lack of sleep and depression are related to low serotonin. It is possible that acupuncture may have some effect on the serotonin levels within the brain.

David Mayer has performed some of the same tests on human beings at the Medical College in Virginia.

Dr. David Mayer at the Medical College of Virginia used normal humans who were subjected to experimental pain caused by electrical stimulation of their teeth. First he showed that

9 P. A. M. Rogers, "Enkephalins," *Acupuncture Research Quarterly*, 1:2 April, 1977, p. 64.

10 *Ibid.*

11 Wang, pp. 78-86.

acupuncture did increase pain threshold. Then he administered Naloxone under double blind experimental conditions. Naloxone significantly reduced the analgesic effects of acupuncture. From this it can be concluded that acupuncture relieves pain by causing a release of enkephalins in the central nervous system![12]

Bruce Pomeranz of the University of Toronto has shown that the electrical activity of spinal neurons is significantly diminished by acupuncture. After removing the pituitary gland from cats, Pomeranz found that acupuncture had no effect on the transmission of pain signals. Since the pituitary is a primary source of endorphin, he concluded that acupuncture needling stimulates nerves deep in the muscles to release endorphin from the pituitary, thereby producing analgesia. The effect of morphine and of endorphin can be blocked by the opiate antagonist, Naloxone.

Pomeranz believes that 30 percent of the patients with chronic pain who fail to respond to acupuncture do *not* have opiate receptors in the brain. This same number of people fail to respond to morphine. About 30 percent of all people cannot be hypnotized, probably the same people who cannot respond to acupuncture or morphine.[13]

THE USE OF AUTOGENIC PHRASES

It once was thought that the autonomic nervous system, which regulates the body's organs, could not be voluntarily or consciously controlled to any significant degree. Recent evidence indicates otherwise. Psychologist Neal E. Miller of Rockefeller University in New York has used a system of reward and punishment to demonstrate that animals can be conditioned to control autonomic processes, such as the flow of blood to various parts of the body.[14]

Human beings also can develop voluntary control of the autonomic nervous system—for example, lowering their blood pressure—apparently by learning to control normally unconscious parts of the mind. This kind of learning usually requires visual or audible feedback, such as a flashing light or a buzzer. These cues inform the subject of his success, telling him if he is controlling what is happening in the normally unconscious domain inside the skin.

[12] Dr. Solomon Snyder, "The Brain's Own Opiates," *Chemical and Engineering News,* Nov. 28, 1977, p. 35.

[13] *Ibid.,* pp. 79-80.

[14] Elmer and Alyce Green, "The Ins and Outs of Mind-Body Energy," *Science Year, 1974: World Book Science Annual* (Chicago: Field Enterprises Educational Corp., 1973), p. 138.

Although there is a line of separation between the conscious and the unconscious, the voluntary and the involuntary nervous systems, this separation apparently can shift back and forth. For example, when we learn to drive a car we focus conscious attention on every detail of muscular behavior and visual feedback. We manipulate steering wheel, gas pedal and brakes according to what we see on the road ahead of us. Visual feedback tells us what we are doing and suggests corrections if, for example, the car heads toward a ditch. Through such feedback we learn conscious control of the striate, or voluntary, muscles. After much experience, driving becomes automatic. We then may take a long drive while thinking about something else and then wonder if we stopped at all the traffic lights.

When this behavior occurs, processes normally controlled by the conscious have temporarily shifted to the unconscious. When, through feedback, voluntary control is exerted over so-called involuntary processes, such as dilating and contracting the smooth muscles that control blood flow, the shift is back to the conscious domain.

Observing the early work in this field, psychologist Gardner Murphy, former head of the Menninger Foundation Research Department, Topeka, Kansas, thought that biofeedback might be useful.[15] This meant connecting monitoring equipment to visual or audible signaling devices. For example, when a thermistor was connected to a meter or a buzzer, the subject could tell if his attempt to change his skin temperature was succeeding by watching the meter needle or hearing the buzzer.

When biofeedback is combined with autogenic training, many people can learn to control unconscious physiological functions more quickly than with either one alone. This combination of the two systems is called "autogenic feedback training." Autogenic training supplies a strong, suggestive imagery and biofeedback supplies immediate knowledge of the results. These are powerful factors in gaining voluntary control of involuntary processes, and are of great importance in continuing research programs.

Many people in the medical profession are anxious to use any biofeedback techniques that will assist the patient in cooperating with the therapeutic program. Many in the medical profession now have biofeedback equipment in their offices. The goal, be it achieved with acupuncture or another method, is for the patient to be able to do his own therapy, leading to the healthiest life possible.

Doctors Alyce and Elmer Green at the Menninger Clinic in Topeka, Kansas, have developed a series of autogenic phrases which

[15] Green, p. 141.

tend to bring the patient closer to the alpha brain wave rhythm. Particularly in situations where tension is a major part of the patient's problem, these phrases can be used by the one giving the massage to the patient:

> You feel quiet; you are beginning to feel quite relaxed; your feet feel heavy and relaxed; your ankles, your knees and your hips feel heavy, relaxed and comfortable; your solar plexus, and the whole central portion of your body, feel relaxed and quiet; your hands, your arms and your shoulders, feel heavy, relaxed and comfortable; your neck, your jaws and your forehead feel relaxed, they feel comfortable and smooth; your whole body feels quiet, heavy, comfortable and relaxed; you are quite relaxed; your arms and hands are heavy and warm; you feel quite quiet; your whole body is relaxed and your hands are warm, relaxed and warm; your hands are warm; warmth is flowing into your hands, they are warm, warm; you can feel the warmth flowing down your arms into your hands; your hands are warm, relaxed and warm; your whole body feels quiet, comfortable and relaxed; your mind is quiet; you withdraw your thoughts from the surroundings and you feel serene and still; your thoughts are turned inward and you are at ease; deep within your mind you can visualize and experience yourself as relaxed, comfortable, and still; you are alert, but in an easy, quiet, inward-turned way; your mind is calm and quiet; you feel an inward quietness.[16]

These phrases can even be recorded on a cassette and given the patient to take home for him to practice relaxation by himself.

It is a well established fact that the patient's emotional reaction to pain must be resolved before pain can be relieved.

Melzack and the Greens have used alpha brain wave feedback training with patients suffering persistent pain.[17] Alpha brain rhythm is associated with feelings of calm. Experiments indicated that patients could relieve their pain by one-third or more, and needed fewer analgesics following autogenic training.

MASSAGE OF PREMATURE AND NEWBORN BABIES

Ruth Diane Rice, a nurse, a psychologist, and a specialist in early child development received her Ph.D. degree from the University of

[16] Originally presented by Dr. Alyce Green at the Menninger Foundation, Topeka, Kansas. Reprinted with permission.

[17] Ronald Melzack, *The Puzzle of Pain,* Basic Books, 1973.

Texas at Austin, after completing a research study in sensorimotor stimulation of premature infants.

Rice developed a specific stroking and massage technique which she used in an experimental study of 30 premature babies. The mothers were taught this technique which includes touching, movement, and the sound of a heartbeat, similar to the conditions the baby experienced in the womb.[18]

Infant research has shown that touching, movement, and sound stimulate the nerve pathways and cause the following to occur:

1.   An increase in myelination, dendritic processes, and Nissl substance in the brain cells resulting in a speeding up of neurological growth.

2.   A higher output of the growth hormone somotrophin, causing faster weight gain.

3.   An increase in the output of the hypothalamus which serves as a general arousal center, leading to increased cellular activity and endocrine functioning.

The development of Rice's stroking and massaging technique and the success she has had using it have brought national and international recognition from persons in medicine, nursing, psychology, and child development.

Rice believes there must be revolutionary changes made in the care of newborn infants and in parent/child interaction if the high incidence of emotional disturbance, learning disabilities, hyperactivity, and many other disorders which have their origins in infancy are to be prevented.

SUMMARY

The recent discovery of endorphins may soon provide answers to the neurophysiological mechanisms involved in relief of pain by acupuncture or massage given to specific areas, such as Bindegewebsmassage. In addition, during massage the use of autogenic phrases will assist the patient to relax. Sensorimotor stimulation by massage facilitates the development of premature infants as well as decreasing the possibility of emotional disturbance.

[18] Ruth D. Rice, "Premature Infants Respond to Sensory Stimulation," *APA Monitor*, 6:11 (November 1975), pp. 8-9.

Part II

The Application of Basic Western Techniques

Chapter 7

General Procedures of Massage

BEGIN CAUTIOUSLY

Generally massage begins with light effleurage which follows the venous flow. Do not massage directly over the most tender areas or the actual site of injury, but proximal to it. As the patient grows accustomed to the touch, the involved area can then be cautiously approached. When the patient can tolerate rather deep effleurage one may work into petrissage. This may be light or deep depending again on the extent of the involvement and tolerance of the patient.

If other techniques such as friction, cross-fiber manipulation, and tapotement are used, they follow the use of effleurage and petrissage. Effleurage is usually interspersed with other strokes and is the stroke ordinarily used to begin and finish a massage treatment.

In concluding the treatment, strokes which work gradually from deep to light should be used. Tapotement, if used at all, is most often given at the end of the massage treatment as a terminal touch. It is not normally used in therapeutic situations unless on stump ends. It is often used in athletic situations or for other stimulation.

USE ORIGINALITY

Judgment and originality must be used to find the correct approach with each patient. In many cases that which "feels good" will be a strong factor in choice of strokes. At other times whether it "feels good" or not, certain techniques will be necessary. Each stroke has a purpose. It becomes the responsibility of the operator to judge from the tissues beneath the working hands which techniques to select; how deep the pressure should be; how gentle the stretching must be; when to progress from one stroke to another; and when to progress from one area to another.

It is never wise to spend too long in one small area. It is more advisable to massage the whole general area, coming back to the areas of tenderness often.

KNOW THE OBJECTIVES

The objective of each treatment should be kept in mind. Each case will have one or more problems, such as pain, limited motion, swelling, etc., which require special attention.

If massage is given for a sedative purpose, the strokes will be slow and rhythmical, using effleurage and petrissage with pressure that is not too deep. Slow, rhythmical effleurage with the part in elevation will reduce edema. If the desired effect is stimulation, speed of the stroke can be increased and deeper pressure can be used.

FOLLOW MUSCLE GROUPS

The operator needs to be aware of the muscle groups involved in each case. The usual procedure is to massage each muscle group (for example the flexors of a joint), applying effleurage and petrissage which can be followed by friction or any other special strokes which may seem indicated. Each muscle group should be "stroked off" with effleurage before proceeding to the next muscle group.

There are times when one may need to approach the involved part by some division other than by muscle groups. The operator may massage the anterior aspect of the body before approaching the posterior in order to avoid asking the patient to turn over more than once. In so doing, the operator should still be aware of the muscle or muscle group that is being massaged.

When muscular tightness is present, friction to the tendons, toward their insertion, will help relieve protective muscle splinting against pain.

Summary

Aside from these general remarks, it is not the feeling of this author that specific instructions can be given for any specific involvement. The operator must be aware of the basic conditions that exist, such as pain, swelling, limited motion, etc., and treat these symptoms, regardless of whether they are caused by surgery, accident, or illness. After learning to apply massage techniques to the various areas of the body, the student will be ready to study the cases in Part IV to learn how to plan individual routines for specific situations.

Chapter 8

Effleurage

Effleurage is used more than any other of the massage techniques. It usually initiates each treatment. The evaluation the operator can make of the patient's soft tissue with this technique can orient him better than a written or verbal report. During these initial strokes, sensitive fingers can explore for areas of tenderness or tightness. Effleurage is often interspersed between other strokes; it is used to progress from one area to another, and is the most common stroke used in concluding the treatment. It should therefore be mastered well, so that it can be performed with rhythm and confidence.

Any stroke that glides over the skin without attempting to move the deep muscle masses is called effleurage. The hand is molded to the part, stroking with firm and even pressure, usually upward.

PURPOSE OF EFFLEURAGE

This stroke is usually used at the beginning and ending of every massage as well as in between all other strokes. It accustoms the patient to the touch of the operator and allows sensitive fingers to search for areas of spasm and soreness. In given instances where extreme soreness is present, it may be the only stroke employed. It serves to distribute evenly whatever lubricant is being used. Deep effleurage will also provide a passive stretch to given muscles or muscle groups. Muscles of the back are illustrated in Figure 8-1.

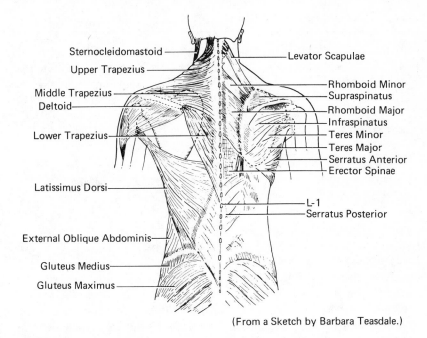

Sternocleidomastoid

Upper Trapezius

Middle Trapezius

Deltoid

Lower Trapezius

Latissimus Dorsi

External Oblique Abdominis

Gluteus Medius

Gluteus Maximus

Levator Scapulae

Rhomboid Minor

Supraspinatus

Rhomboid Major

Infraspinatus

Teres Minor

Teres Major

Serratus Anterior

Erector Spinae

L-1

Serratus Posterior

(From a Sketch by Barbara Teasdale.)

Figure 8-1. Muscles of the back.

POSITION OF EFFLEURAGE TO THE BACK

First see that the patient is comfortable, lying prone with the feet either off the end of the treatment table or supported at the ankle by a roll or pillow. A pillow under the abdomen is often a good idea and the arms may be placed wherever they are most comfortable. The head may be turned to either side.

In cases where it is difficult for a patient to lie down and get up, he can be treated in a sitting position. If this is done, he can rest his arms and head against the treatment table and they can be supported by pillows if necessary. Naturally, he must be seated on a stool or sideways on a chair so that the back can be free for treatment.

DRAPING FOR MASSAGE TO THE BACK

The patient is asked to loosen or remove any clothing that might interfere with the massage. This can be done after he has been covered with a sheet. If he needs assistance it should be given when he asks for it or if the operator notices that he needs assistance. It is usually easier for the patient to loosen all clothing before turning to lie prone. The operator then pulls the sheet down to the level of the coccyx, being careful not to expose the gluteal cleft. The sheet can be tucked over the edge of the patient's clothing or pajamas in order to protect them from the lubricant. This draping will suffice for these early practice techniques. If the low back is involved the entire gluteal area should be massaged. This is discussed more thoroughly in Chapter 13.

APPLICATION OF EFFLEURAGE TO THE BACK

Since powder leaves a clear pattern to follow, apply it using enough so a pattern can be seen when learning this stroke. Remember that too much powder will prevent good contact between the hand and the skin. Place both hands on the patient's back at the level of the coccyx, with the heel of the hand close to the spine and the fingers pointing outward. Make sure the whole hand is relaxed so that the entire palmar surface touches the patient's body. Allow the hands to glide slowly along the erector spinae group, being careful to avoid the spinous processes. As the neck is approached, the hands move upward to the base of the skull.

The return stroke downward may have lighter pressure progressing laterally, with the fingers molding over and in front of the shoulder to encompass the whole upper trapezius. As the stroke progresses, it follows the fibers of the upper trapezius to the shoulders and thence down the latissimus dorsi to the upper half of the gluteals. (See Figure 8-2.)

Effleurage may be light or deep depending on the amount of pres-

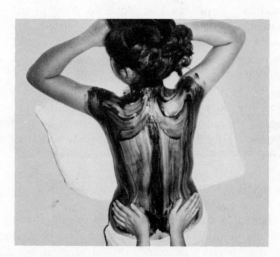

Figure 8-2.   Fingerpaint pattern of effleurage.

sure applied, but this pressure should be the same throughout the stroke, until the student learns more about how to vary it.

Points to check while practicing:

1. Is the patient *comfortable?*

2. Is the patient *relaxed?*

3. Are the *hands* of the operator relaxed?

4. Is pressure even throughout each stroke?

5. Is the stance one of good body alignment, with weight over feet, or has the weight been allowed to fall forward over the treatment table?

6. Is *all* of the hand in contact with the patient?

7. Look at the powder patterns on the patient's back. Compare them with Figure 8-2.

VARIATIONS OF EFFLEURAGE

Whenever the pressure of any effleurage stroke over any part of the body is light, it is referred to as *light effleurage* regardless of the part of the body to which it is applied or the pattern that may be followed.

By the same token, any effleurage wherein the pressure is deep is referred to as *deep effleurage*. Stroking and effleurage are terms that may be used synonymously.

The student should attempt to make his pressure light throughout the entire stroke and again deep for the whole stroke. If he can do this well he may then try to let his pressure start light and increase until it is quite deep, tapering off again until it is quite light at the end of the stroke. The student should then ask the "patient" to guide him by telling him which pressure feels best, remembering that this "patient" is not one with an injured or arthritic back, but an essentially healthy one.

Knuckling is a stroke particularly associated with the techniques of Hoffa. In describing it he says:

> If the part to be treated is covered by thick fascia, effleurage is not deep enough. You need greater pressure, therefore the convex dorsal sides of the first interphalangeal joints must be used. Clench the fist in strong palmar flexion; the peripheral end of the knuckles should be upwards. Gradually bring the hand from plantar to dorsal flexion. Pressure is not continuous, but swells up and down, starting lightly and becoming stronger, then decreasing

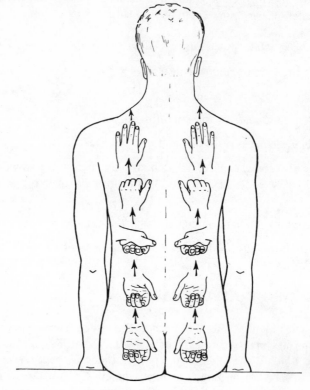

Figure 8-3.   Application of knuckling stroke.

again in pressure. The hand must not adhere to the part but should glide over it lightly. Knuckling should only be used where there is enough room for the hand to be applied [see Figure 8-3].[1]

Shingles refers to an alternate type of stroking in which one hand follows the other with the strokes overlaying themselves one after the other like the shingles on a roof. Thus, although contact with the patient is lost as each hand is lifted, the remaining hand maintains contact, giving the patient a feeling of constant contact.

Bilateral tree stroking refers to both hands progressing simultaneously on either side of the back, from the spine laterally, and upward with short strokes that build like the branches growing from the trunk of a tree.

[1] Albert J. Hoffa, *Technik der Massage*. Stuttgart: F. Enke, 1900, p. 2. Translation by Frances Tappan and Ruth Friedlander.

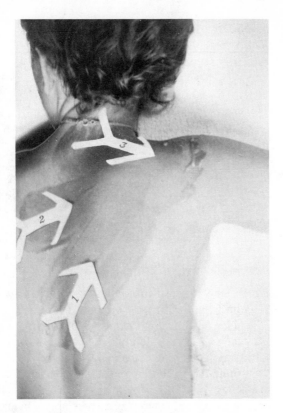

Figure 8-4. Three-count stroking of the trapezius.

Three-count stroking of the trapezius (Figure 8-4) can be done with a rhythmical three-count stroke which begins at the origin of the lower trapezius, progressing with one hand toward the insertion. Simultaneously, the other hand moves to the origin of the middle trapezius where it begins its stroke just as the first hand concludes, progressing toward the insertion of the middle trapezius. As soon as the first hand has completed its stroke of the lower trapezius, it progresses *without contact* to the origin of the upper trapezius and strokes downward to the insertion to complete the third part of this three-count routine. This particular method of stroking the whole trapezius is rhythmical and relaxing when well done, but it must be timed like the shingles strokes so that, in spite of the lost contact, as each hand is raised, the patient feels constant contact because one hand is always stroking.

Horizontal stroking is particularly useful when applied to the low back. Place both hands lightly on the patient's back as shown in Figure

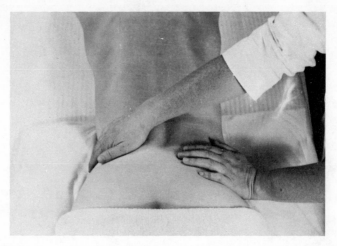

Figure 8-5. Horizontal stroking to the low back.

8-5. Using a stroke similar to effleurage, move the right hand forward and the left hand backward with firm pressure. When the hands have gone as far to the sides of the patient as possible, the stroke direction is reversed *without* changing the position of the hands. As the hands return to their original position a strong *lift* and *push together* of the hips is executed. The returning hands continue all the way over to the opposite side of the patient, thus going from side to side across the back. No pressure should be placed over the spinous processes as the hands pass over them. Greatest pressure comes into the *lift* and *push together* of the low back as the hands pull upward and inward to meet and cross over the spinous processes and continue on down each side of the patient. This feels especially good to the patient who has a sacroiliac involvement.

Mennell's superficial stroking can be distinguished from light effleurage by its unidirectional flow "going either centripetally or centrifugally but never in both directions," and by its return stroke through the air which must be "controlled as for rhythm" taking as long as that part of the stroke which contacts the patient. Only the lightest possible pressure is used in this stroke.[2]

Concluding stroke for relaxation is used if preparing the patient to relax for sleep. The treatment is concluded with long, light, effleurage strokes which start at the base of the skull, stroking directly over the spinous processes, going all the way down to the coccyx. Pressure must

[2] Mennell, pp. 24-27.

be very light but firm and the rhythm monotonous; pressure that is too light would stimulate rather than sedate. As one hand is about to complete the stroke near the coccyx, the other hand begins the next stroke starting at the base of the skull, giving the patient the feeling of continuous contact, with one hand beginning the next stroke before the other finishes. If this technique is kept up for a minute or two it helps the patient relax completely. The patient often obtains a tingling sensation throughout the arms and legs which facilitates relaxation. Some patients will even fall asleep before the treatment is finished. If this technique is applied beyond two or three minutes it tends to stimulate rather than relax so it should never be continued for long.

SUMMARY

The effleurage strokes most often used in America today have been discussed. They should not limit the creative person who wishes to develop other types of effleurage strokes to suit the individual needs of a patient. Neither should he be restricted in adjusting the strokes described here on the back to all other parts of the body. The study of petrissage will teach the student how to combine these two massage techniques. While learning petrissage, effleurage should be interspersed between petrissage strokes for two reasons: to provide practice for the student, and to prevent "over petrissage" on any part of the body.

Chapter 9

Petrissage

Petrissage is difficult to describe, but not difficult to perform. Contrary to effleurage which glides over the skin, petrissage strokes attempt to lift the muscle-mass and wring or squeeze it gently. Care should be taken not to work in one area too long before progressing to the next and not to pinch or bruise the tissues. These strokes should be practiced on the back until they can be done rhythmically and with good close contact before being attempted on other parts of the body.

Petrissage consists of kneading manipulations which press and roll the muscles under the hands. It can be done with one hand, where the area to be kneaded is small, or it can be done with two hands on larger areas. It can even be done with two fingers on very small areas. There is no gliding over the skin except between progressions from one area to another.

PURPOSE OF PETRISSAGE

This kneading motion of petrissage serves to "milk" the muscle of waste products which collect due to abnormal inactivity. It assists the venous return and in given instances it will also help to free adhesions.

Position and draping for application of petrissage to the back would be the same as that for effleurage (see Chapter 8).

TWO-HAND PETRISSAGE TO THE BACK

Since all petrissage is preceded by effleurage as a preliminary stroke, review the effleurage strokes, first stroking lightly and then working gradually into a deep effleurage.

Now place both hands firmly on one side of the patient's back, with the lower hand ready to start its motion over the upper portion of the gluteals.

Although each hand is going to describe a circle, counter-clockwise in direction, they do so with such timing that as one hand moves away from the spine across the muscles of the back, the other hand is moving medially toward the spine (see Figure 9-1). The hands are almost *flat* as they shape themselves to the contours of the back. They pick the tissues up *between* the hands (not *with* the hands), and as they "pass" each other the forceful part of the stroke is executed as the muscles are pressed downward against the ribs and rolled between the hands.

After about three repetitions of this stroke in one position, progress upward by allowing the lower hand to slide up to where the top hand has just been working, as the top hand glides upward to a new position.

Petrissage does not require much lubricant. The hands should cling to the part being massaged, picking up and pressing, sliding only when progressing, and even then with enough pressure so that fluids in the tissues are carried along with the stroke.

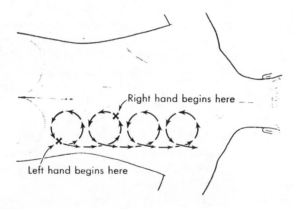

Right hand begins here

Left hand begins here

Figure 9-1. Petrissage of the back.

VARIATIONS OF PETRISSAGE

Alternating two-hand petrissage to the back

This type of petrissage for the back is very useful for following the direction of muscle fibers such as the trapezius.

Alternately use the index and middle fingers of one hand working with the thumb of the other hand. The thumbs are placed one above the

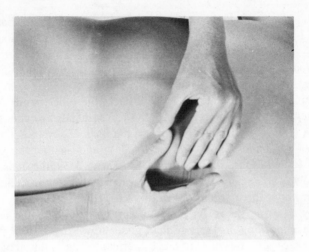

Figure 9-2. Alternating two-hand petrissage to the back.

other (see Figure 9-2) and remain in this position, although the emphasis of each stroke is carried first by one hand and then the other. The fingers of one hand reach proximally, pick up the muscle, and move toward the opposite thumb. At the same time the thumb is pressing toward the proximal aspect of the muscle, moving toward the fingers. The opposite hand then repeats this same motion, and both hands alternately work from distal to proximal aspects of the muscle group.

Two-Finger Petrissage on Broad Flat Areas

Following the erector spinae muscle group up the back, grasp a small part between the thumb and first finger. Press it out as is done in other petrissage strokes. Although the movement is small, the whole motion should come through a relaxed arm.

Other variations of petrissage are best practiced on areas smaller to grasp. Positioning and draping are described in Chapter 13 with the discussion of massage to the upper extremity. For purposes of this early practice they can be referred to briefly.

When applying any of the following techniques to areas of the body other than the back, "C" and "V" positions of the hand are used.

The C and V position names are derived from the C-like formation of the hand position as it grasps the arm or leg with the thumb in abduction and slightly flexed with the fingers cupped to fit the part being massaged. Pressure is exerted on the palm and the palmar surface of all fingers according to the contour of the part (Figures 9-3, 9-4). The wide or open C would be applied to the hand position where a large area such as the thigh is involved (Figure 9-3). The narrow, or closed C (Figures 9-4, 9-5) refers to the use of the same position when it is applied to an arm or smaller area. On very narrow areas the position is so narrowed that the thumb comes into adduction and the position is then referred to as the V position (Figure 9-6).

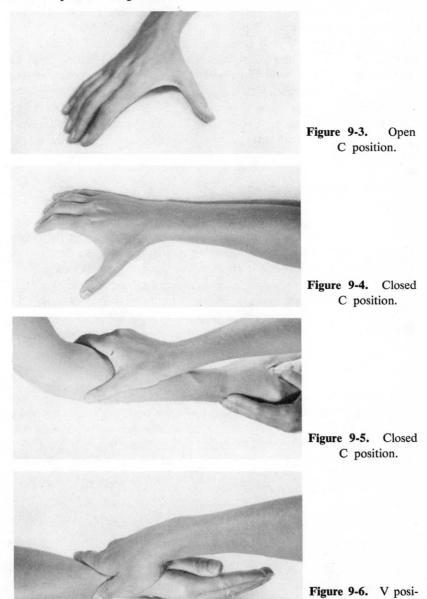

Figure 9-3.   Open C position.

Figure 9-4.   Closed C position.

Figure 9-5.   Closed C position.

Figure 9-6.   V position.

One-hand Petrissage

For use on smaller limbs (arms and children's legs) one hand is sufficient for petrissage. Place the hand *around* the part, picking up the muscle mass, using the *whole* hand. Lift the muscle away from the bone, squeezing gently upward and making small circular motions. Let the hand relax on the downward part of this small circle.

As with the two-hand petrissage, the rhythm should be slow and regular. Progression upward to a new position should follow three or four strokes. As the hand progresses, pressure is upward, carrying the venous return and lymph with it.

Since the biceps offers a distinctive, easily-grasped muscle, apply one-hand petrissage to the upper arm. Let the muscle belly fit into the palm of the hand while the thumb and fingers apply pressure to the upward part of the stroke.

Alternate One-Hand Petrissage

Another approach to petrissage of the upper arm may be accomplished by grasping the biceps in one hand and the triceps in the other. Using an alternate pattern of squeezing, petrissage both the flexors and the extensors with a soothing rhythm. As the one hand is relaxed, the other is putting on pressure with the same, upward, circular strokes.

In circumstances where a certain amount of stimulation is indicated, this stoke can be used to advantage, progressing rather rapidly with each stroke working always in the direction of the venous flow.

Summary

Other variations of petrissage are included in Part III. These fine differences should not be attempted until the basic approach has been mastered. Later, if the operator can do one technique better than the other, he can then be selective in the technique he prefers. While learning friction, both effleurage and petrissage should be interspersed, since people practicing on each other often work too deeply and bruise the tissues.

Chapter 10

Friction

Although massage could consist of only effleurage and petrissage, friction is necessary to reach beneath the more superficial tissues. Storms and Cyriax think that friction is the most important massage technique and base most of their massage treatment around this stroke.[1] When used correctly it permits the operator to work into the deeper tissues gradually, judging how far to go by the patient's reaction.

Friction is performed by small circular movements with the tips of the fingers, the thumb, or the heel of the hand, according to the area to be covered. Small flat ellipsoids are described which penetrate into the depth of the tissue, not by moving the fingers on the *skin* but by moving the tissues *under* the skin.

PURPOSE OF FRICTION

Friction is used to massage deep into the joint spaces or around bony prominences such as the patella. It is especially useful around a well-healed scar to break down adhesions between the skin and tissues which are beneath it. It *cannot* affect a deep fibrositis such as might form within a muscle belly.

---

[1] Harold Storms, "Diagnostic and Therapeutic Massage," *Archives of Physical Medicine,* Vol. XXV (September 1944), pp. 550-52.

APPLICATION OF FRICTION TO THE BACK

Arrange the patient as for a back massage and begin the treatment with effleurage and then petrissage.

Using the ball of each thumb, place one on each side of the spinous processes of the back (see Figure 10-1). Any level of the back will do for a spot to learn the technique. Press as deeply as the patient can tolerate without pain, describing small circles with a force that comes down through the arm from the shoulder. These small circles do not slide across the skin (as effleurage does), nor do they "pick up" or "squeeze" (as petrissage does). They gradually press into the tissues, becoming deeper as the patient develops tolerance to the pressure. Pressure should never be released suddenly.

Progress upward after about three cycles, following bilaterally upward to the side of the spinous processes, and in the muscular spaces between the transverse processes. The student learning friction should never practice too long in one spot because his attempts to obtain deep pressure may cause bruising until he learns his own strength and adjusts his technique.

Pressure follows up either side of the spine, avoiding the bony prominences. Following deep friction, effleurage stroking of the immediate area may be done with the thumbs to help the patient relax.

While the thumbs are doing the major portion of the work with this technique, the rest of the hand rests lightly on the back. It does not brace the thumb.

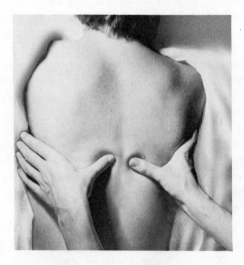

Figure 10-1.   Friction.

VARIATIONS OF FRICTION

Cross-Fiber Manipulation

Deep friction-like strokes which apply pressure *across* the muscle fiber, rather than along the longitudinal axis of the muscle fibers, can be applied to the erector spinae group of the back. Unlike typical friction strokes the thumb moves across the skin with deep short strokes.

Place one thumb close to the spinous process and stroke outward with deep pressure. Follow this stroke immediately by doing likewise with the other thumb, working thus, alternately up the back.

This type of manipulation can be done over any localized area, particularly in the presence of nodules or localized tightness.

Storms' Technique

Harold D. Storms of Toronto, Canada, developed a stroke which he used both for diagnostic and therapeutic measures, particularly for fibrositic nodules.

The cushions of the fingertips or the ball of the thumb do not slide over the skin; instead, they hold position on the skin, the short stroke being made possible by moving the connective tissue *under* the skin.

This stroke varies from the previously described friction strokes in that the direction of the stroke is always parallel to the muscle fibers, rather than circular or cross-fiber in direction. Storms specifies also that as soon as the spasm *begins* to soften, massage should stop for that day.

Cyriax's Friction for Fibrositic Muscles

Cyriax recommends deep friction given to the site of the lesion, which may or may not be within the painful area outlined by the patient.

There are four ways in which one may use his hand to provide friction *across* the fibers of the structure being treated. Muscle, ligament, and joint capsule require friction administered perpendicularly to the long axis of the fibers composing them. The thicker and stronger the tissue, the greater the exactitude needed.

This can be done using the index finger crossed over the middle finger; using the fingertips of the middle and ring fingers; using opposed fingers and thumb in a pinching position; or by using the superimposed thumbs, with the one thumb reinforcing the other.

SUMMARY

Although there may be times when friction is not used at all in giving massage, there are other times when effleurage and petrissage merely prepare the tissues for the deeper application of friction. If one concentrates on working into this depth *gradually*, the patient will be able to tolerate more depth. By the same token when the operator is "letting go" it should be gradual and slow so that the patient experiences no sudden change. The following discussion of tapotement will further develop the student's knowledge of massage technique. As previously stated, all techniques learned thus far should be interspersed in practice of tapotement since, until one has mastered the art of "bouncing off," the patient may take a slight "beating."

Chapter 11

Tapotement

Although tapotement is not used as often as the other massage techniques, it does have its place and requires practice to be able to perform it well.

Because of the indiscriminate use of tapotement in beauty salons and as often shown in motion pictures on prizefighters, and because of the unscientific claims that excess flesh can be "beaten off," many operators shun using it at all. It should not, because of this misuse, be ignored. If anything, emphasis on doing it correctly, and definition of its proper use, should be stressed.

Any series of brisk blows, following each other in a rapid, alternating fashion, come under the broad term of tapotement. Included under this heading are hacking, cupping, slapping, beating, tapping, and pincement.

PURPOSE OF TAPOTEMENT

Tapotement is used when stimulation is desired. Since most massage is for purposes of relaxation, tapotement is often not a part of the general routine of massage. In athletics where stimulation is usually the purpose of massage it plays a more important role. Occasionally the apathetic patient may receive slight stimulation and a pleasant sensation of well-being following masasge which has been terminated with tapotement.

APPLICATION OF TAPOTEMENT TO THE BACK

Hacking

Before reading the following instructions, shake the hands, letting the wrist, hand, and fingers relax and "flip up and down." No attempt should be made to hold the fingers together or the hands or wrists in any particular position. If relaxation is complete, it will be noticed that the hands fall into a neutral plane of motion which neither supinates nor pronates the forearm (see Figure 11-1).

When relaxation is complete, an alternate direction of each arm can be started. One moves up as the other moves down, still keeping the hands relaxed and shaking them (see Figure 11-2).

Approach the patient, holding the hands so that the palms are parallel. Strike the back with a series of soft, but brisk blows, using the backs of the third, fourth, and fifth fingertips. Use both hands, alternating them and striking rapidly (Figure 11-3). Done correctly the effect is one of *pleasant* stinging and stimulation.

Progress from the hips upward to the shoulder and then back downward to the hips again. Tapotement should never be done over the kidneys. For an increased stimulation effect, use alcohol applied with one or two rapid, light effleurage strokes just previous to the hacking strokes.

Cupping

This stroke is applied with the same rhythmical, rapidly alternating force, changing only the position of the hands to apply the blow with a cupped hand. Cup the hand so that thumb and fingers are slightly flexed, and the palmar surface contracted (see Figure 11-4). Strike the

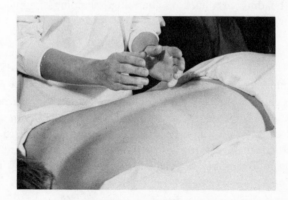

Figure 11-1.   Starting position.

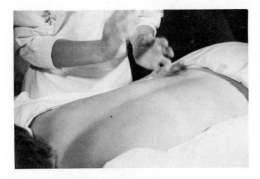

Figure 11-2. In motion.

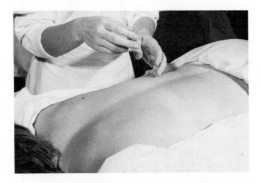

Figure 11-3. On contact.

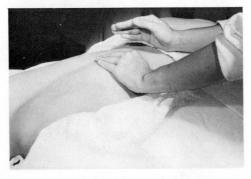

Figure 11-4. Cupping.

back with the palm of the hand. This presumably causes a slight vacuum with each blow and some people believe it may loosen the broad flat areas of scar tissue. It makes a rather loud noise if done correctly, which could be detrimental or useful, depending on the psychological situation at hand.

Slapping

In the same manner, but using an open rather than a cupped hand, strike gently but briskly with the fingers, rather than the palm of the hand (see Figure 11-5).

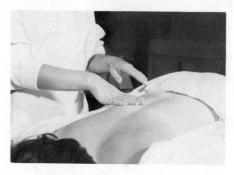

Figure 11-5. Slapping.

Beating

The same stroke can be done using the hypothenar eminence of the hand, with the fist closed. Care should be taken to keep the force of the blows light and "bounding" in effect rather than jarring (see Figure 11-6).

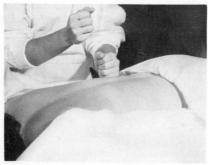

Figure 11-6. Beating.

Pincement

Likewise, rapid, alternate, *gentle* pinching that picks up small portions of tissue between the thumb and first finger can be done (see Figure 11-7).

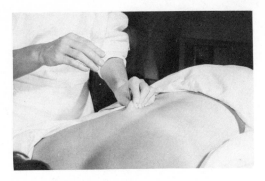

Figure 11-7. Pincement.

Tapping

Tapping is done with the ends of the fingers, using sharp taps that make use of moderate fingernails, or padding the tap by using the pads of the fingers if the patient cannot tolerate the sharpness of the ends of the fingers.

SUMMARY

Any series of brisk blows following each other in a rapid alternating fashion come under the broad term of tapotement. They may be hacking, cupping, slapping, beating, tapping or pincement. The purpose is usually to provide stimulation. These techniques need much practice to be applied with skill and if one cannot do them skillfully they should not be used at all.

Chapter 12

Vibration

Vibration was developed in Europe. Although it is described here for those who want to use it, it is this author's opinion that vibration can be given better with an electrical vibrator, with the exception of the very gentle vibration mentioned in treating peripheral neuritis and poliomyelitis.

A fine tremulous movement, made by the hand or fingers placed firmly against a part, will cause the part to vibrate.

PURPOSE OF VIBRATION

Vibration is often used for a soothing effect, particularly in treating peripheral neuritis. The treatment follows the path of the nerve. Vibration for this purpose must be very gentle and rhythmical, using fine vibrations. It has been used in Europe for poliomyelitis patients with such delicacy that the vibrating hand does not even touch the part, but merely flutters above it.

APPLICATION OF VIBRATION TO THE BACK

Use the same draping and position previously described. Place one hand anywhere on the back with the fingertips slightly apart. The rhythmical, trembling movement comes from the whole forearm, through the elbow, but the wrist and finger joints are kept stiff. The elbow should be slightly flexed. This vibrating motion should be more up and down, than side to side. Heavy pressure should be avoided, especially if used with peripheral neuritis patients.

VARIATIONS OF VIBRATION

When following the path of a nerve for a soothing effect, an effleurage type of stroke done with just the fingertips is employed, adding the vibration to the light effleurage stroke. Pressure can even be made so light that there is almost no contact of the hand with the part, and the vibrating hand moves almost out of contact. With extremely hypersensitive cases this technique has been credited with bringing a soothing effect.

Shaking

Another variation of vibration in a much coarser degree is useful for patients who have difficulty relaxing. If often helps to pick up the muscle belly (especially the biceps or gastrocnemius) and gently shake it back and forth. It is also helpful at times to shake the entire limb gently in order to encourage relaxation.

SUMMARY

Vibration should not be used at all if one has not put the time and effort into learning to do it well. Done well it can be extremely soothing, but done poorly it will only cause frustration and impatience on the part of both patient and operator. It is difficult to learn well, and seldom used in America. Emphasis given to this technique must be decided by the operator.

This concludes the basic strokes of massage. The following chapters describe how these techniques can be applied to any part of the body for therapeutic effects.

Chapter 13

Application to Parts of the Body

As previously emphasized, each patient will display different symptoms even though the diagnosis for different patients may be the same. The following suggestions pertaining to each of the different areas of the body point out some general approaches that make it easier for the operator to apply massage. Trained, sensitive fingers searching for muscle spasms, nodules, tightness, and painful areas should be able to locate the unique symptoms of each patient.

MASSAGE OF THE BACK

Using the positions and draping described in Chapter 8, effleurage and petrissage should be given to the following muscles or muscle groups:

Erector spinae	Trapezius
Latissimus dorsi	Rhomboids
Gluteals	Levator scapuli

Light effleurage to all of the above will make the operator aware of tense or painful areas to be given more detailed consideration later in the treatment. All strokes should follow the muscle fibers. Any or all of the techniques learned previously can be applied. A variety of strokes and patterns can be selected to treat the individual complications that each patient may have.

MASSAGE OF THE LOW BACK

Position

When positioning the patient for a low back involvement, the operator should consider putting the spine in slight flexion by placing a pillow under the abdomen with the patient face-lying. Some patients cannot lie comfortably in this position. If moving is difficult or impossible, the operator must adapt the techniques so that the patient can be treated side-lying or even lying flat on the back. Therefore, effleurage and petrissage should be practiced with the "patient" lying in all positions. This involves applying the strokes at different angles. Consequently, the operator may find the height at which he has been working needs to be adjusted by stepping on or off a low platform.

When lying on one side, the patient should have the top leg well supported. The top arm should be supported in a position where the operator is sure the patient is not using it to help maintain the side-lying position. Pillows under the leg and arm will not only give them support, but also will keep the patient from falling forward when pressure is applied to the back.

Draping

Draping is no different in principle for any of these positions. A sheet or towel should keep any part that is not being treated covered and warm.

Application of Technique

Because of heavy fascia in the low back area, many patients can tolerate rather heavy pressure. The piriformis is often in spasm and only deep friction through relaxed gluteals can exert any pressure on it. The amount of direct mechanical pressure which can be applied on this muscle is debatable.

MASSAGE OF THE GLUTEI

Many people will be sensitive to massage of the glutei, therefore some special approaches should be discussed.

Draping

As little of the area should be exposed as possible. Only that which is necessary should be left uncovered. The operator can often work under the sheet. If only one side is involved a sheet can be placed so it covers the entire other half of the body, including the gluteal cleft.

Application of Technique

The operator can help the patient adjust to the touch of his hands by working on either the lower extremity or the back, stroking gradually toward the gluteal area. This is contrary to the usual approach of massaging the proximal area first. The purpose of reversing this procedure is to help the patient adjust to treatment of this area.

Strokes to this area need to be heavy due to the large muscle-mass. They should follow the direction of the muscle fibers for each of the gluteal muscles. Follow the usual sequence of effleurage, petrissage, and friction where indicated. Deep effleurage strokes which go around the acetabulum and the tuberosity of the ischium should be included. It is difficult to reach through this large muscle-mass to palpate the piriformis which is often in spasm, but with relaxation of the gluteals it can sometimes be accomplished.

Friction can often be tolerated about the lumbosacral and sacro-iliac regions but should be done carefully since these areas are often sensitive. Friction should also be done over the area of the greater sciatic notch, the ischial tuberosities, and the area between the iliac crest and the greater trochanter and around the greater trochanter.

If the patient must lie on his back, the problem for the operator is to reverse the technique from applying pressure downward to that of reaching under the patient and applying pressure upward. Effleurage is fairly easy to do in this fashion but petrissage is much more difficult. One hand can effect the circular motion of the usual two-hand petrissage, progressing up the back. Friction is also easy to apply, using the tips of the fingers with the palm facing the patient, working with the typical small circles of friction or with a cross-fiber technique.

Practice of massage to the back should be done with the "patient" in all positions, even seated with the head resting on a pillow against the treatment table, because patients with back involvement often find lying down very difficult.

MASSAGE OF THE CERVICAL AND THORACIC SPINE

Position

Patients requiring massage of the thoracic or cervical spine are often more comfortable lying face down, with a pillow under the chest, and with the head supported by a small, rolled towel in a neutral position. Patients have a difficult time getting comfortable if they have pain in this area. One often discovers that the patient is better at finding a comfortable position for himself than being told in which position to lie. If it is impossible to find a comfortable position lying down, the massage can be given with the patient in a sitting position, leaning on a pillow placed on the treatment table. Either position is acceptable. Possibly the sitting position is a little more convenient for the operator. The arms may be placed wherever comfortable as long as they do not support the weight of the patient and are relaxed. In some instances the head may be held supported with a Sayre head sling for support or slight stretching combined with massage. Some patients will be more comfortable in a back-lying position with the operator standing at the head of the treatment table.

Draping

There should be no clothing on the upper back. Women may be given a hospital gown which splits down the back but protects the rest of the body if treated in a sitting position. If the patient is lying down, the draping is the same as it has been for the other techniques applied to the back.

Application of Technique

All of the variations of effleurage described previously can be applied to this area. The three-count stroking of the upper trapezius (Figure 8-4) is especially useful. Stretching can be applied to the upper trapezius. Use one hand to stabilize the head and the other to give a deep effleurage stroke which goes from the origin to the insertion of the upper trapezius. Pressure should be deep enough to stretch the muscle fibers but never deep enough to cause pain. Care should be taken that the stabilizing hand does not push the head away. It maintains good alignment of the cervical spine, serving to hold the head still so that the stretch is accomplished by pushing the shoulder downward, not by pushing the head away.

Sayre Head Sling and Stretching

In cases where the Sayre head sling has been prescribed, effleurage strokes for the upper trapezius can be applied while the patient is receiving traction from the head sling.

Care should be taken to see that pressure is so placed that normal alignment of the cervical spine is not displaced.

Verbal instructions for relaxation will assist the patient in getting maximal benefit from this type of treatment (see autogenic suggestion phrases, Chapter 6).

All petrissage techniques can be adapted to this situation, even the one-hand petrissage, which can be used on the upper trapezius. Two-hand petrissage can also be done on the muscle-mass of the upper trapezius, which can be grasped with the hands molding over the anterior aspects of the muscle. If deep petrissage is done with upward progression toward the head, it should be followed by deep effleurage strokes downward to assure good venous return. Watch the complexion of the patient; if the face is flushed, only downward pressure should be used.

Friction may be used as previously described (Chapter 10), following up the spine on either side of the spinous processes all the way up to the occiput. Any involvement of the upper back or neck is apt to cause marked tenderness at the occipital protuberance. Friction, therefore, is cautiously applied around the tendinous insertion, or not done at all if the patient cannot tolerate this type of pressure.

Mennell refers to "sensitive deposits" which can be felt under the exploring hand of the operator.[1] These deposits are often found in the muscle bellies in this area and can be treated as described by Mennell or Storms. Storms' methods have already been discussed (Chapter 10). Mennell advocates the use of frictions that begin gently at the periphery of the sensitive area and gradually approach the center of it. This should be followed by deep petrissage. Cross-fiber manipulation may also be used in a similar fashion.

Although *tapotement* and *vibration* may be used, these strokes are not routinely part of the treatment.

MASSAGE OF THE CHEST

Position

The patient should be back-lying with due consideration for the relaxation of all muscles that originate or insert from the chest. Slight flexion at the knees would tend to relax the abdominals. Pillows under the arms will relax the pectorals. A pillow under the head should relax the muscles of the neck.

Draping

A towel or sheet should cover the side not being treated to keep the patient warm and comfortable.

[1] Mennell, p. 474.

Application of Technique

Any or all of the techniques described, except tapotement, may be applied to the chest. Because of the many types of surgery or injuries that could be treated in this area, no particular approach to special muscle groups can be outlined. Involved muscles should be treated by groups. Scar tissue and limited shoulder movement, especially following mastectomy, may often be the major concern. Stretching should be applied if the shoulder has been held in protective splinting which leads to tightness. In this event consideration should be given to those posterior muscles that may also be tight.

MASSAGE OF THE ABDOMEN

Position

The patient should be back-lying with the knees in slight flexion and supported so that the hip flexors and abdominal muscles are relaxed. The head may be resting on a pillow.

Draping

A towel or sheet should cover the upper part of the patient, and another one the lower part of the patient so that only the abdomen is exposed.

Application of Technique

Orders are almost never received for abdominal massage. There was a time when it was ordered for constipation. This author does not recommend it, but includes it for those who might want instruction.

Gentle effleurage strokes should be used to accustom the patient to the touch of the operator. All strokes should follow the direction of the colon, as it ascends on the right, crosses, and then descends on the left. Gradually increase pressure (but never too heavily). Light petrissage may follow the same pattern followed again by effleurage.

It is usually easier for the operator to stand on the patient's right side.

Friction, with precaution against going too deeply, can then follow. Use circular strokes that follow the direction of the colon. Complete the treatment with light effleurage in the same direction.

Caution: Abdominal massage could cause serious complications in the event of pregnancy, appendicitis or other abdominal disorders.

MASSAGE OF THE UPPER EXTREMITY

Position

Range of motion in the shoulder joint may be the deciding factor as to whether the patient will be treated in a sitting or lying position. If there is tightness of the pectorals, but not inhibiting pain, it is well to treat the patient sitting with the arm supported. This puts a slight stretch on tight muscles while the patient is being treated. The amount of stretch can be increased by raising the height of the arm or lowering it if it cannot be tolerated. If severe pain, as with bursitis, prevents this position, the arm may rest on a pillow in the patient's lap or on a lower table. Some patients are more comfortable lying down.

If the hand or wrist is involved, the hand is usually supported by a small roll or towel, so that it rests with the wrist slightly extended. The fingers, if relaxed, will rest in partial flexion. This position also puts the fingers slightly off the table, which protects the fingertips from bumping on the table if they are hypersensitive.

Draping

Only the arm being treated should be left uncovered. A towel or a sheet may be used to cover the patient in such fashion that it will not slip, especially if the patient is in a sitting position. If the entire arm is to be treated, the draping should cross the shoulder not being treated and be fastened securely with a safety pin. Sleeves of the patient should never be pushed up. The shirt or blouse should be taken off to prevent tight clothing from inhibiting the venous return.

Application of Technique

The greatest change noticed in adapting the strokes to the arm and hand is in the position of the operator's hand. As previously described, the hand is open to cover the wide surfaces of the back. On the arm and hand a closer position will be used to encompass the smaller area with close contact, using either the C or the V position.

Upper Arm

Muscles or muscle groups to be considered in massage of the upper arm would include those of the cervical and upper back if the shoulder is involved. (See pages 70–71 for general procedures.) These muscles are often tense from muscle splinting to avoid pain in the injured or involved arm. If so, they should also be treated. Muscles of the arm include the pectorals, serratus, deltoid, triceps, and biceps. In addition to massage for each muscle or muscle group, the joints should be considered. Care should be taken not to place deep pressure into the joint or over bony prominences.

Elbow and Forearm

The patient is seated. The arm rests on a pillow, providing flexion of the elbow and pronation of the forearm. Give two short strokes toward the insertion of the biceps, first the medial side then the lateral side. Stroke from distal to proximal along the medial border of the upper third of the brachioradialis. Stabilize the elbow joint from the back. Follow the upper third of the ulnar side of the palmaris longus stroking toward the origin. Stop before the epicondyle. Give long stokes that pull from the distal two-thirds of the brachioradialis. Change hands.

Give long strokes on the ulnar side of the palmaris longus, beginning at the lower third of the arm and stopping at the epicondyle. Change hands.

Stabilize the wrist. Pull over the ulnar border of the flexor carpi ulnaris. Stop before the condyle. Stroke on the dorsal side of the arm along the edge of the extensor digitorum communis from the lower third of the origin. Bimanual "widening" of the elbow joint is done with the patient's elbow flexed. Hold the olecranon and pronator teres in one hand, and the brachioradialis in the other hand Pull outward with both hands (Figures 13-1 and 13-2).

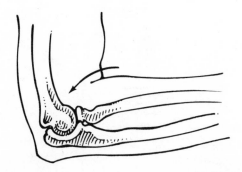

Figure 13-1. Lateral view of stroke to elbow.

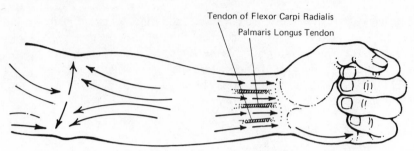

Figure 13-2. Application of massage to the elbow and forearm.

Lower Arm

In the lower arm the flexors of the wrist and fingers can be treated as a group. The extensors comprise the other major muscle group to be treated. Those muscles which cross both the elbow and the wrist should be considered. Both of these joints should be included in the massage and any limited range of motion should be *gently* stretched using effleurage strokes which encourage increased range of motion.

If some of the muscles of the upper arm, such as the biceps, are involved due to muscle splinting or casting positions, the massage should include treatment of them also.

Application of Technique

To perform massage strokes the operator uses the soft pad of any finger, pulling with some depth from distal to proximal.

As illustrated in Figure 13-2, the first stroke pulls over the lower third of the flexor carpi radialis. The second stroke pulls over the palmaris longus. The third stroke pulls over the flexor carpi ulnaris (Figure 13-3).

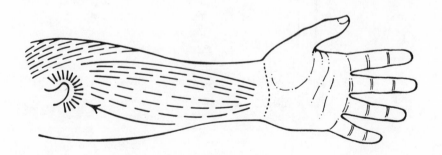

Figure 13-3. Stroking the Palmaris Longus.

Hand

A common problem of an inexperienced operator is the *over-stretching* of the capsule in the small joints of the fingers. The fingers need to be stretched *gently*. A gentle, steady pull, combined with slow effleurage wherein the operator's first finger surrounds most of the finger, while the thumb covers the dorsal aspect, will feel good and also be beneficial to the patient. However, the "popping" of the joints can be very harmful and should be avoided. A Mennell type of passive motion, which gently encourages active motion and increases the range of motion, can be combined with massage of the fingers. *Little good can come from overstretching.* It tears the tissues and causes increased swelling and pain.

The fingers are so small that massage is difficult. It must be practiced until it can be done well. Hand injuries are common and the swelling and limited motion that accompanies such injuries need treatment.

All strokes previously described can be adapted to these smaller areas and must be mastered. Elisabeth Dicke's strokes so completely cover all aspects of massage to the hand that they are included under Bindegewebsmassage (see Chapter 17). For general massage the author prefers that all strokes proceed from distal to proximal, while Dicke describes strokes from proximal to distal.

MASSAGE OF THE LOWER EXTREMITY

Position

The person receiving massage to the lower extremity should be lying down with the leg in a neutral position or elevated in the event of swelling. There should be support at the knee and at the ankle. The foot should never be allowed to drop into plantar flexion, even though it is not necessarily involved. A pillow or drop-foot board should support the foot at about 90 degrees of dorsiflexion.

The person may be face-lying if most of the treatment pertains to the posterior aspect of the leg. In this case the feet should be off the end of the treatment table and the lower leg supported so that the knee is in slight flexion, unless stretching of the hamstrings or gastrocnemii is indicated.

Draping

With an injured lower extremity it is often difficult for the patient to get out of pajamas or trousers. This can easily be handled by asking the patient to loosen the top of his pajamas or trousers. Then advise him to hang onto the top of the sheet. Standing at the foot of the bed, reach under the sheet and pull the trousers off. Always check to be sure the patient has a tight hold on the sheet or both the sheet and trousers will come when the trousers are pulled.

Occasionally there is demand for what is jokingly called "diaper" draping (Figure 13-4). This can be tactfully managed by handing the patient a towel and asking him to place it so that it goes between his legs, covering him, both front and back. He can do this while protected by the sheet, working under it, or the operator can leave the room while the patient drapes himself.

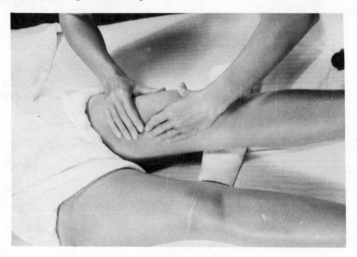

Figure 13-4. "Diaper" draping. Massage to the upper leg.

Application of Technique

Mold the hands to the contours of the leg in applying effleurage and petrissage to the muscle groups involved. Care should be taken not to carry any strokes too high on the medial thigh. All of the principles mentioned in massage of the upper extremity also apply to the lower extremity.

Upper Leg

Muscle groups that should be considered in massage of the upper leg include the gluteals if the hip is involved. The hamstrings, adductors, abductors, and quadriceps should be treated as groups and are

usually involved in injuries to the hip or knee, or fractures of the thigh.
The hip flexors are seldom massaged, but in the event of hip-flexion contractures they would benefit from treatment.

Gentle stretching of the hamstrings and gastrocnemius may be
done. Using both hands just above the popliteal space, lightly hold the
tendons of the hamstrings with the fingertips. Lift and supinate both
hands, gently stretching the tendons (Figure 13-5). This same technique
can also be used for the two heads of the gastrocnemius, just below the
popliteal space, but never working deep into the popliteal area.

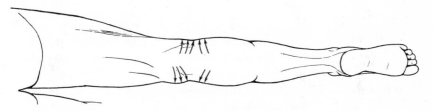

Figure 13-5.   Application of massage to the upper leg.

In cases of injuries to the leg, the patella often lacks normal
mobility. In cases of arthritis care should be exercised so as not to
work too deeply with friction around the patella. Use one hand to
stabilize the patient's leg, while using the other hand to perform short,
deep friction-like strokes that follow the border of the patella (see
Figure 13-6).

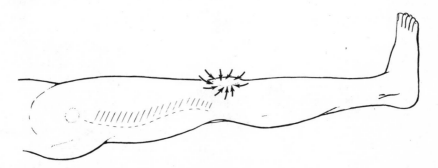

Figure 13-6.   Friction-like strokes to the patella.

Pivot-like strokes, in which the heel of the hand acts as a pivot
and the fingers stroke around the borders of the patella, can also be
used (see Figure 13-7).

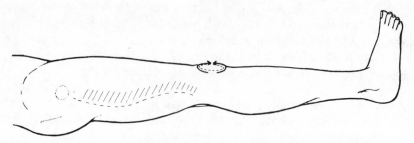

Figure 13-7.   Pivot-like strokes to the patella.

Lower Leg

In the lower leg, the tibialis anterior, tibialis posticus, the peroneals, and the gastrocnemius comprise most of the muscle masses which are to be treated as muscle groups. These muscle groups can be effleuraged and petrissaged in preparation for detailed attention to be given to any particular problems.

Use bimanual stroking of the Achilles tendon, working from distal to proximal, from the medial and lateral malleolli upward over the gastrocnemius. The hands flex the foot slightly as they stroke (see Figure 13-8).

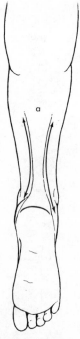

Figure 13-8.   Stroking to the Achilles tendon.

Stroke the peroneus longus and brevis, around the malleolus, and proximally up the leg. Stabilize the leg with one hand.

In the same fashion, stroke the tibialis posticus and around the malleolus (see Figure 13-9a). Complete the series by stroking bimanually both of these areas at the same time.

Foot

All of the principles brought out in the discussion of massage to the hand, particularly the special care taken when working with small joints, apply to massage of the foot.

Stabilize the foot with one hand. Use little strokes moving distal to proximal across the front of the ankle joint. Dorsiflex the ankle while stroking (see Figure 13-9b).

Apply short small strokes between the metatarsophalangeal joints, going from distal to proximal, then medial to lateral (see Figure 13-9c).

If the toes are involved they will be massaged exactly as the fingers.

Deep short strokes should be made just in front of the heel, from the arch along the side of the foot, starting laterally and working medially. The same thing should be done going the other way, starting medially (see Figure 13-9d).

Short strokes can be made across the bottom of the heel. Deep stroking of the plantar fascia can be done with long strokes which cover the longitudinal arch from the heel up to the metatarsophalangeal joint, using the knuckles to achieve deep pressure (see Figure 13-10). Foot reflexology will be discussed in Chapter 18.

Plantar stroking may also go across the muscle fibers at right angles to the longitudinal arch (see Figure 13-10b).

Bilaterally stretch both the top and bottom of the foot with a rolling motion of the hands; up and out on the proximal part of the

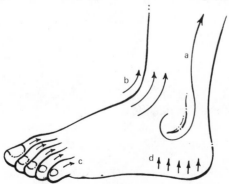

Figure 13-9.   Massage to the lower leg and the foot.

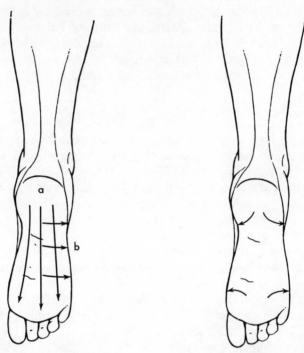

Figure 13-10. Plantar stroking across muscle fibers.

Figure 13-11. Bimanual stretching of the foot.

foot. On the distal part of the foot, reverse direction to stretch the forefoot (metatarsal arch) in the opposite direction (see Figure 13-11).

MASSAGE OF THE FACE

Position

The patient may be lying down or seated, as preferred. The operator stands behind the patient.

Draping

A small towel or head band may be used to keep the hair away from the face during the treatment.

Application of Technique

In cases of Bell's Palsy the involved side of the face is often stretched, being pulled by the well muscles on the opposite side, especially around the mouth. In giving treatment, both sides should

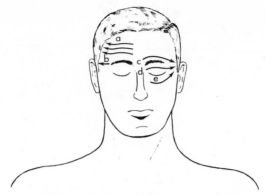

Figure 13-12.   Massage to the face.

be massaged, since the side of the face *not* paralyzed will also have muscles that are tight. Support to lessen this pull should be given with the hand not being used to massage, alternating as both sides are treated.

Bimanually stroke across the forehead, from the hairline down to just above the eyebrows, moving from the center of the forehead toward the temple (Figure 13-12a).

Stroke gently using the pads of the fingers from the lateral side of the eye into the hairline of the temple (Figure 13-12b). Follow the upper eyebrow, stroking from medial to lateral toward the temple (Figure 13-12c).

Repeat the same, following the lower rim of the eyebrow (Figure 13-12d).

Repeat the stroke just below the eye (Figure 13-12c).

Apply short strokes upward between the eyes (Figure 13-13a).

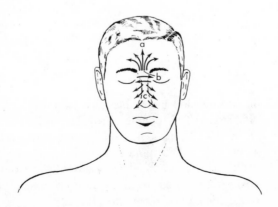

Figure 13-13.   Massage between the eyes.

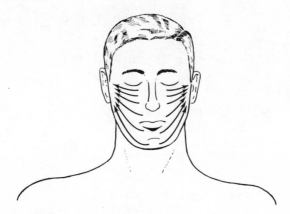

Figure 13-14. Stroking the zygomaticus.

Pull from the involved side to the uninvolved side over the bridge of the nose. Reverse the direction (see Figure 13-13b).

Bimanually stretch the nose, stroking from the center to each side. Work all the way down to the very tip of the nose (see Figure 13-13c). Bimanually stroke the zygomaticus, working from just under the eyes toward the mandible, stroking from front to back (see Figure 13-14). Soft strokes directly over the closed eyes of the person, pulling from the nose lightly over to the temple, can be very relaxing.

Petrissage can be performed with two fingers in the smaller areas and with the thumb opposing the fingers over the fleshier parts of the face.

Gentle friction directly over the temples is especially good for a headache. Friction all around the hairline will ease tension caused by frowning or muscle tightness that originates there. With finger and thumb, the bridge of the nose can be stretched by pulling it outward.

For all of these strokes, gentleness must be emphasized, and care taken not to put pressure directly over the eyes. Contact lenses should be removed.

SUMMARY

Each person will develop his or her own combinations of strokes for all parts of the body. This chapter provides many suggestions to assist the learner in developing skill in adjusting the hand, whether the area is large or small. The hand can more easily be studied in Chapter 17, in which Dicke's method is discussed. The author, however, prefers strokes to proceed from distal to proximal instead of from proximal to distal as in Dicke's procedure.

Chapter 14

Use of Massage in Nursing and Physical Education

MASSAGE BY NURSES

The development of therapeutic touch is central to nursing because the nurse with trained and sensitive hands can greatly enhance the quality of patient care. Dolores Krieger has demonstrated in controlled studies the positive physiological effects of touch [1] (see Chapter 5). Furthermore, through the "laying-on of hands" one can communicate the uniquely human *concern* of one individual for another, in an act that incorporates an intent to help or heal the person so touched.

Massage provides a valuable approach that can comfort the distraught patient if the nurse applying the treatment extends her concern, both verbally and tactilely. The patient may literally feel the interest and compassion extended for his welfare.

With skillful hands the nurse can gain the confidence of her patients. Discomfort can be relieved and positive attitudes developed. Physiological, mechanical, and reflex effects can also be accomplished. Such a massage need not take more than five minutes. In fact, more than five minutes may do more harm than good.

Patients confined to bed develop areas of physical discomfort due to inactivity. Chapter 13, Part I, explains the physiological reasons

---

[1] Dolores Krieger, "Nursing Research for a New Age," *Nursing Times*, April 1976, p. 1.

for this discomfort and tells how massage can relieve this type of distress.

Any or all of the techniques described in this book may be used. Massage of normal tissues, which is not involved with the patient's pathological condition, can often relax him when he is restless from long hours in bed. Nurses who can skillfully execute basic massage techniques will earn the gratitude of their patients.

Massage of the Back

If the patient has been lying on his back for quite a while, massage to the back is recommended. In preparing the patient for rest and sleep, the entire massage should be done in a slow, rhythmical, relaxed fashion. This contact presents an excellent opportunity to build confidence in the patient and promote feelings of security and well-being. While empathy can be shown without words, a soothing voice, combined with light rhythmical stroking, can also strongly motivate the patient toward restful sleep.

Muscular tightness through the shoulder and neck muscles due to uncomfortable resting positions and increased tension in the patient can be relieved with strong petrissage to this area.

In concluding, strokes should work from deep to light. Strokes which go downward from the head toward the coccyx are more restful than those which go upward. The relaxing stroke described in Chapter 8 will often leave the patient almost asleep.

Massage for Pressure Areas

Patients who lie quietly in bed due to paralysis or weakness, should receive good massage to areas where pressure is apt to cause decubitus ulcers. Combined with frequent changes of position and proper resting positions, massage can help prevent their formation.

Deep strokes which bring blood to the area should be applied each time the patient is moved. Here again, this need not take a great deal of time, but the results are most gratifying.

Common sites for decubitus ulcers are over the sacrum, the back of the heels, elbows, and knees. When the patient is turned one can readily see where pressure has recently been placed. Effleurage and petrissage may be applied with depth. Stroking *toward* the pressure areas will encourage capillary dilatation. Friction can also be applied around the pressure area. Once a decubitus ulcer has developed to an acute phase, massage alone will be of little use and should not be attempted by the nurse.

Massage for the Immobilized Patient

Patients who have been immobilized by traction or casts often become uncomfortable because of positions that must be maintained. The patient with a leg in traction may complain that his back or neck is uncomfortable.

With precaution against moving the injured limb, massage to the uncomfortable area can relieve much of this discomfort.

USE OF MASSAGE IN ATHLETICS

The well-rounded training program of any physical education major should include massage. The coach should know how to make use of massage for conditioning before activity, and how to prevent or reduce lameness following extreme activity. This does not mean that all athletes could be given a conditioning massage before every game.

There are apt to be instances when massage might help some outstanding member of the track or swimming team break a record. In such cases, massage might add extra nourishment to the vital muscle groups to make this extra effort worth the coach's time.

Massage for Conditioning Before Extreme Activity

Treatment should be given the day before the expected activity. The athlete should plan on a half hour of complete rest following this treatment and an evening that insures minimal exertion and a good night's sleep.

Massage should be preceded by a brisk needle shower, from warm (about 110° F; 45° C) to cool (80° F; 25° C).

With the person lying prone, give a brief general massage which covers the back. Work from light effleurage rather quickly into deep effleurage and petrissage of all the large muscle groups of the back. Encourage relaxation and make sure that the resting position is comfortable.

When sufficient general relaxation has been obtained, massage can be begun on the muscle groups that will be used most in the activity planned for the coming day. Thus, if the event requires running, the legs would be carefully massaged with deep effleurage of the gluteals, hamstrings, and gastrocnemii, working to deep kneading of all these muscle groups, not forgetting the anterior aspects of the leg, particularly the quadriceps and anterior tibial group.

When each muscle group has been carefully massaged, the whole extremity should be gone over again with long sweeping effleurage strokes which follow from the heel all the way up the back of the leg and over the gluteals.

Brisk tapotement of any type leaves the patient with a feeling of tingling well-being.

In the same manner, if the coming event involves the arms, the latter part of the massage should consider mostly the thoracic spine and arms. If the activity involves the use of all four extremities, the total body should be considered, doing first one side and then the other.

Those who have had experience have come to realize the value of putting essential muscle groups into a good metabolic state previous to extremes of activity. There is less tendency toward charley horse with such conditioning, and less tendency toward lameness following the activity.

This concept is far from new. It has been used since the days of the ancient Roman gladiators.

Massage Following Extreme Activity

Whereas the purpose of preconditioning is to ready the muscles for exertion, the purpose of massage following such activity is to carry away the waste products which have collected due to this exertion. It does not require stimulation, for the muscle has been stimulated and is now tired, and seeks rest and inactivity. If the muscle is exhausted enough, it will not perform its normal activity of "milking" these by-products into the venous return. The person who has put forth a supreme effort is physically tired, and at this stage exercise cannot accomplish the desired exchange in metabolism because the muscles themselves are too weary to profit by further exercise.

Therefore, the purpose at this point is to "wring out" the muscle and mechanically do this job of milking for it. Gently kneading the muscle free of such by-products will allow it to take advantage of the fresh supply of blood and lymph which automatically follows the massage.

Since stimulation is not desired, a warm shower should precede the massage. The rate of the stroke is much slower. (Remember the flow of lymph is slow and sluggish.) Watch the more superficial veins and give them time to refill following the effleurage stroke. If muscle soreness is involved, pressure must be regulated so that it is firm enough to squeeze out the muscle without provoking a "muscle splinting" type of protective tensing.

Tapotement is not indicated unless the individual requests it, for now the aim is not one of stimulation or preparation, but rather, rest and complete relaxation. This in itself allows a normal return of new and nourishing blood to the tired muscle and minimizes the tightness and spasm that come from stiff and sore muscles.

If any tightness or spasm is present, and there is no injury to the muscle, such as rupture or hematoma, active normal range of motion may be attempted. If there has been any sign of injury to the muscle, no treatment of any kind should be attempted without consultation with a physician.

Charley Horse (Muscle Cramp or Spasm)

If a muscle is asked to do more than it has been "conditioned" to do, and extreme activity is undertaken without proper warm-up exercises or a building-up to be able to do a task of sudden activity, the result will be sudden, painful spasm of the muscle. The muscle is not able to meet the chemical exchanges to keep its metabolic balance.

The name *charley horse* has also been given to the painful spasm that results from severe kicks or blows, which are accidentally received in competitive activity.

Upon occasion the muscle will actually rupture and hematoma can readily be seen. If there is any indication that these spasms or cramps have been severe enough to cause bleeding within the muscle belly or tearing of the tendon, no measures should be taken to massage or exercise the part until advised to do so by a physician.

If, however, there is cramping due to inability of the muscle to meet the metabolic needs and stresses placed upon it, effleurage and petrissage can assist the muscle back to normalcy. If the muscles do go into spasm, it is an indication that these muscles are not in condition for activity. Conditioning exercises will avoid repetition of such "casualties."

SUMMARY

General knowledge of all the massage techniques will be valuable information for those in the field of physical education. Precautions should be taken to avoid massaging any injury that should not be treated by these techniques. The major uses of massage in athletics presented in this chapter will lessen chances of injury, prevent unnecessary lameness, and prepare muscles for peak performance.

Massage of the back is useful for the patient who has been lying in one position for quite a while. Pressure areas should be massaged to prevent decubitus ulcers. Patients who have to be immobilized by traction or casts develop specific areas of discomfort that can be relieved by massage.

Recent research indicates the importance of extending *truly caring attitudes* from one human being to another. Massage given by a caring person can enhance the quality of patient care because physiological, psychological, and reflex effects can be accomplished by the "laying-on of hands." Attitudes of compassion can be expressed through massage, even if only for five minutes of a nurse's time.

Part III

Variations of
Massage Techniques

Chapter 15

Finger Pressure
to Acupuncture Points

HISTORY OF ACUPUNCTURE

Although the origin of Chinese medicine is lost in antiquity, it is assumed to have developed from folk medicine. It has many aspects in common with other Oriental traditions, such as Indian herbal medicine and Persian medicine. The origin of acupuncture, however, is unique to the Chinese branch of Oriental medicine.

The earliest known text on acupuncture is the *Nei Ching,* or *Classic of Internal Medicine*, traditionally ascribed to the legendary Yellow Emperor (Huang Ti, supposed to have lived 2697–2596 B.C.). Still extant, the *Nei Ching* remains the basic reference on the subject and is the foundation for all developments in acupuncture to the present century.

The ancient Chinese became aware of an increased sensitivity of certain skin areas (called points) when a body organ or function was impaired. It was observed that in all patients the same skin areas became hypersensitive in the presence of a specific illness or organ dysfunction. Consequently, some of the relationships between various internal organs and their functions were observed and established. These were defined and explained in terms of a complex philosophical hypothesis that attempted to relate all the observed phenomena.

Acupuncture has a known history antedating Christianity by 2,000 years. Over the course of centuries a long line of ancient practitioners, belonging to a people noted for meticulous visual observation, were able to establish the existence of a number of meridians and their relationships with various physiological functions. Fundamental to the concept of meridians in Chinese medicine is not only their function as imaginary lines linking a series of points on the skin that become sensitive in the presence of organic or functional disorders, but also their function as actual "energy pathways." The Chinese word for energy is *chi*.

This energy is considered to circulate throughout the body in a well-defined cycle, moving in a prescribed sequence from meridian to meridian and from organ to organ, flowing partly at the periphery and partly in the interior of the body. Like the Western concept of "nerve-energy potential" or the *prana* (life force) of Indian philosophy and medicine, *chi* is a dynamic force in constant flux.

Acupuncture was introduced to the West in the seventeenth century by Jesuit missionaries sent to Peking. Since that time several attempts have been made to promulgate this therapy in the Orient, with varying degrees of success. Not until the French sinologist and diplomat Soulié de Morant published his voluminous writings on acupuncture in the 1940s did Western physicians have a sound basis for study and application of this ancient system of healing.

Under the impetus of de Morant's work, acupuncture associations and study groups were established in many Western countries, among them France, Italy, Britain, West Germany, Argentina, and the Eastern European nations. Many countries now actively support research programs in the physiology and application of acupuncture, notably the U.S.S.R., the People's Republic of China, North and South Korea, and Japan.

Acupuncture is not only presently the focus of growing interest in the West, but it is also undergoing a resurgence of serious study in the Far East. In China, acupuncture is now an integral part of the nation's medical practice, and an increasing number of press reports reaching the West outline some of its more startling applications.

The field of acupuncture treatment is that of impaired body functions, as opposed to actual lesions. In the case of a patient with diabetes, for example, if there is no actual tissue degeneration in the islets of Langerhans, acupuncture can be extremely effective. Even if lesions have formed and are well established, the pain, discomfort, and other symptoms caused by them are greatly relieved by acupuncture. It is impossible, however, to obtain complete and lasting relief of a functional problem that has an organic substratum by use of acupuncture.

One of the primary functions of acupuncture is to directly affect the energy level, and therefore the functioning, of the internal organs by either stimulating or depressing their actions.

MERIDIANS—A MYSTERY?

Oriental philosophy and medical science believe that meridians are a system of pathways, or channels. The meridian system provides for a continuous flow of vital energy and nutrients to all parts of the body. Although there seem to be neither definite anatomical meridian structures throughout the body, nor a specific relationship to existing systems as we know them, Robert Tsay observes that the ". . . meridian system may differ somewhat from the nervous system, the blood circulation and the endocrine system, but it is also possible that it is intimately related to these three systems." [1] The theory of the meridians is the basis for diagnosis and treatment. According to Tsay, ". . . it is impossible for the physician to differentiate symptoms, or to prescribe accurately the exact treatment for a patient without using this theory as a guide or basis. This is the reason it is necessary for the student of Chinese medicine to first study the theory of the meridian system. It is as important as the student of Western medicine having to first learn anatomy, physiology, and pathology." [2]

The 12 regular meridians are, with rare exception, listed in the order of vital energy and nutrient flow as follows:

1.	(L) Lung	7.	(UB) Urinary Bladder
2.	(LI) Large Intestine	8.	(K) Kidney
3.	(St) Stomach	9.	(P) Pericardium
4.	(Sp) Spleen	10.	(TW) Triple Warmer
5.	(H) Heart	11.	(GB) Gall Bladder
6.	(SI) Small Intestine	12.	(Liv) Liver

(GV) Governing Vessel, and (CV) Conception Vessel, the first two extra meridians, are the thirteenth and fourteenth of the most used meridians.

(GV) covers the total posterior midline of the body and a midline portion of the head anteriorly. (CV) covers the remaining anterior midline portions of the head and body.

As listed, circulation of energy and nutrients starts through (L), continuing through each of the meridians in succession. From (Liv) the

---

[1] Robert C. Tsay, *Textbook of Chinese Acupuncture Medicine, Volume One, General Introduction to Acupuncture* (Wappinger Falls, N.Y. and Las Vegas, Nev.: Assoc. of Chinese Medicine and East-West Medical Center, Ltd., 1974), p. 44.

[2] Tsay, p. 52.

energy flows to and through the (L) meridian again. The complete cycle takes 24 hours and repeats continually throughout life. Branches of the meridians allow for the vital energy transport from one meridian to the other.

Features of the Meridians

No real anatomical "vessels" can be found by dissection. Two components of circulation go through the meridian circulatory system: *Chi*, the invisible circulation of the vital energy; and *Hseuh*, the visible circulation, including blood and lymph.[3]

Meridians are named according to: (1) the organ that is controlled by the energy flow, i.e., lungs, stomach, spleen; (2) the function of the energy, i.e., Governing Vessel, Regulating Channel, and Motility Channel; and, (3) Yin or Yang.

In a Yin meridian, energy mainly flows upward. In a Yang meridian, energy mainly flows downward. The Oriental Yin and Yang theories compare in some ways to what Western scientists call positive and negative elements, which exist in every atom. Even when atoms are split, particles still maintain positive and negative charges. Only very recently have scientists thought that anything at all could exist without a positive and a negative particle.

The Oriental philosophy believes that the solar system is a large universe with its Yin and Yang. All lives are part of it, and the human body is like a smaller universe within this particular galaxy. Since an atom contains its Yin and Yang, a cell therefore contains its Yin and Yang, and an organ contains its Yin and Yang. Any individual body that may be deemed a unit must also contain its Yin and Yang.

Upon review of the literature on meridians, one will find that various authors name the system differently. For example, meridians may be called channels or pathways. The meridians may also be named in other ways, e.g., Lung, (L), is also Pulmonary, (PU); Large Intestine, (LI), is also Colon, (C); Stomach, (St), is also Gastric, (GA).

There are the following types and numbers of meridians: (1) 12 regular meridians; (2) 8 extra ones; (3) 12 chief branches and 12 muscle branches; (4) 15 liaison vessels; (5) 12 cutaneous liaison vessels. The 14 meridians most often used are the 12 regular ones and the two extra meridians, Governing Vessel, (GV), and Conception Vessel, (CV).

As vital energy and nutrients flow during the 24-hour cycles, there are two-hour intervals when a maximum of vital energy is reached in

---

[3] Tsay, pp. 40-41.

each of the 12 regular meridians. Intervals start with 0300–0500 in the Lung meridian. This maximum vital energy time is considered the best time to treat pathologies of that meridian. As McGarey [4] points out,

> If asthma attacks occur, particularly at night, it is felt best to treat the problem during that two-hour period between three o'clock and five o'clock A.M. In the Western world, it does not seem likely that this would get done outside an emergency room very often, but, nevertheless, this is the rule of acupuncture and should be recognized as such for whatever value it may have at some future time in one's experience.

Flow in the meridians follows three specific cycles within the 24-hour period. Each cycle contains four meridians, as grouped within the 12 meridians. Figures 15-1 through 15-8 illustrate the four meridians in each cycle, with the direction of the flow indicated. Figures are shown with upper extremities raised above shoulder height to better illustrate the *up* and *down* direction of the vital energy and nutrient circulation. In each figure the right side is used as the right side in both anterior and posterior views. Remember, the meridians are bilateral, therefore the circulation is duplicated on the left.

A total of 20 enlarged dots are located on the meridians in all but one of the figures (Figure 15-3). These indicate acupuncture points, each named according to the meridian on which it is located. The 20 points have been selected by specialists in the field. They are thought to be most effective when used, in various combinations, for treating common painful areas, i.e., head, shoulder, low back, and leg. Selection was made from the 642 points found on (1) the 14 most used meridians —361; (2) Special Acupuncture Points, also called Extra Points—171; and (3) New Acupuncture Points—110.[5]

Each of the three cycles illustrated has the following features: each cycle is composed of four different meridians; each meridian is either a Hand or a Foot meridian; each is either a Yin or a Yang meridian; and each has a two-hour interval when a maximum of vital energy is reached, called the maximum energy time. Each cycle also has a definite sequential direction of vital energy and nutrient flow through the four meridians of that cycle. Flow starts through a Yin meridian, going *up* from the chest area to the *hand*; then from the *hand*, *down* toward the chest and

---

[4] William A. McGarey, *Acupuncture and Body Energies* (Phoenix, Arizona: Gabriel Press, 1974), p. 35.

[5] Huang, Min Der, Medical Seminar at Chinese Acupuncture Science Research Foundation, Taipei, Taiwan, R.O.C. 1975.

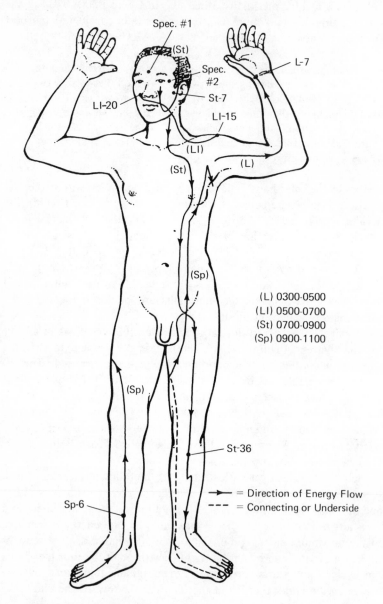

Figure 15-1.   First cycle anterior.

head area via a Yang meridian; from the head area *down* a Yang meridian to the *foot*; and then from the *foot*, *up* to the chest area via a Yin meridian. Then flow continues to the next cycle Yin meridian in the

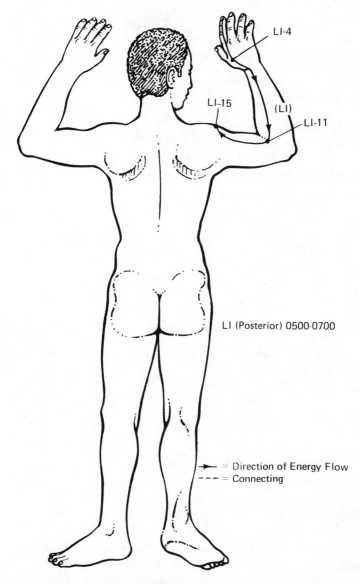

LI-4

LI–15

(LI)

LI-11

LI (Posterior) 0500-0700

→— = Direction of Energy Flow
--- = Connecting

Figure 15-2. First cycle posterior.

chest. Features of the three cycles are included in Table 15-1.

Governing Vessel (GV) and Conception Vessel (CV), the thirteenth and fourteenth of the most used meridians, are illustrated in

Table 15-1

MERIDIAN (ABV.)	HAND OR FOOT	YIN OR YANG	MAXIMUM ENERGY TIME	FLOW: UP, OR DOWN	POINTS LOCATED ON FIGURES
1. FIRST CYCLE (FIGURE 15-1) ANTERIOR					POSTERIOR (FIGURE 15-2)
(L)	Hand	Yin	0300-0500	UP	(L) 7
(LI)	Hand	Yang	0500-0700	DOWN	(LI) 4, 11, 15, 20
(St)	Foot	Yang	0700-0900	DOWN	(St) 7, 36
(Sp)	Foot	Yin	0900-1100	UP	(Sp) 6
					Special Points #1, #2
2. SECOND CYCLE (FIGURE 15-3) ANTERIOR					POSTERIOR (FIGURE 15-4)
(H)	Hand	Yin	1100-1300	UP	
(SI)	Hand	Yang	1300-1500	DOWN	(SI) 3
(UB)	Foot	Yang	1500-1700	DOWN	(UB) 40, 60
(K)	Foot	Yin	1700-1900	UP	
3. THIRD CYCLE (FIGURE 15-5), ANTERIOR					POSTERIOR (FIGURE 15-6)
(P)	Hand	Yin	1900-2100	UP	(P) 6
(TW)	Hand	Yang	2100-2300	DOWN	
(GB)	Foot	Yang	2300-0100	DOWN	(GB) 20, 21, 30, 34
(Liv)	Foot	Yin	0100-0300	UP	(Liv) 3

Figure 15-7 and Figure 15-8. The former also shows the combined posterior acupuncture points while Figure 15-8, (CV), shows the combined anterior acupuncture points. For example, (GV) 26, one of the 20 most used acupuncture points, is seen on Figure 15-8.

Meridians are connected, in couples, through 15 points, called Lo Meridian Points. Liaison vessels serve as links between coupled meridians. As Tsay describes them, "Coupled meridians, composed of a Yin meridian and a Yang meridian, are closely interrelated as an inseparable body. Three couples are on the hand, and three on the foot. Couples may evidence identical symptoms, and can be treated at the same meridian points." [6] (Meridian and acupuncture points refer to the same points.)

[6] Tsay, pp. 78-79.

The meridian system is built anatomically in a nonspecific system functioning to balance all aspects of the human body: mental, digestive, reproductive, nerve, and circulatory processes; internal and external organs; energy, nutrition, and consciousness. Tsay notes, "Viewing meridians as lines—it is possible to see that many meridian pathways run closely parallel to the pathway of one or more main nerve branches. The anatomical relationship of the bi-meridian points with blood vessels are (sic) also very close, but not as close as with the nerves." [7] In order, then, to understand the workings of the body, to recognize symptoms of dysfunction, and to prescribe treatment, persons studying Chinese healing arts need the same basic knowledge of the meridian system as those persons studying Western healing arts need anatomy, physiology, and pathology.

PHYSIOLOGY OF ACUPUNCTURE

Studies proving that the electrical excitability of nerves can be reduced by acupuncture needles *only* have been done on animals and man (see Chapter 6 for a discussion of Dr. David Maver's work).

In 1975, Dr. Frederick Kerr, Department of Neurologic Surgery at Mayo Clinic in Rochester, Minnesota, reported a study he conducted using rats.[8] The first rat was given acupuncture to Ho-Ku, Large Intestine 4. This reduced its trigeminal nerve excitability by 75 percent. The second rat was given no acupuncture, but was given a blood transfusion from the first rat with an acupuncture needle in his Ho-Ku. The result was that the second rat showed considerable lowering of excitability in its trigeminal nerve.

It has been shown that acupuncture points can be located with electrical apparatus, and that electrical resistance of the skin is consistently lower at acupuncture points. Acupuncture point areas often are tender, small nodules. Moreover, temperature differences in acupuncture points have been demonstrated with infrared photography.[9]

Needling sites also seem to correspond with the "Head Zones" discovered by Sir Henry Head in the 1800s. Pain resulting from pathology of the viscera is often referred to clearly definable areas on the body surface known as "Head Zones." These zones closely relate to the twelve acupuncture meridians and are associated with the same organs.[10]

[7] *Ibid.*, p. 61.

[8] Frederick W. L. Kerr, M.D., in a conference at the University of Connecticut Health Center, September 29, 1975.

[9] McGarey, p. 11.

[10] M. E. Armstrong, "Acupuncture," *American Journal of Nursing*, September 1972, pp. 1582-88.

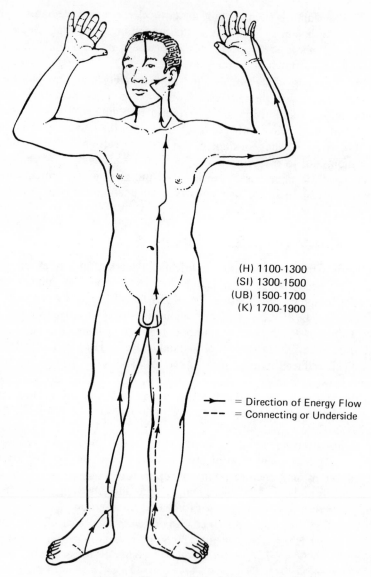

(H) 1100-1300
(SI) 1300-1500
(UB) 1500-1700
(K) 1700-1900

→ = Direction of Energy Flow
--- = Connecting or Underside

Figure 15-3. Second cycle anterior.

Organs receive their autonomic nerve supply primarily from the homolateral part of the nervous system. Connective tissue changes can therefore be found on the corresponding part of the body surface. The liver, gall bladder, duodenum, ileum, appendix, ascending colon, and hepatic flexure receive their nerve supply mainly from the right. The

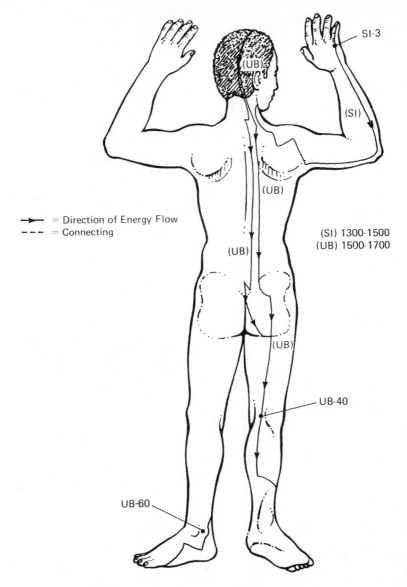

SI-3

(SI)

= Direction of Energy Flow
= Connecting

(SI) 1300-1500
(UB) 1500-1700

UB-40

UB-60

Figure 15-4. Second cycle posterior.

heart, stomach, pancreas, spleen, jejunum, transverse and descending colon, sigmoid colon, and rectum receive their nerve supply mainly from the left.

Changes relating to the bladder, the uterus, and the head can be found in the middle of the back. Changes relating to the lungs, bronchi,

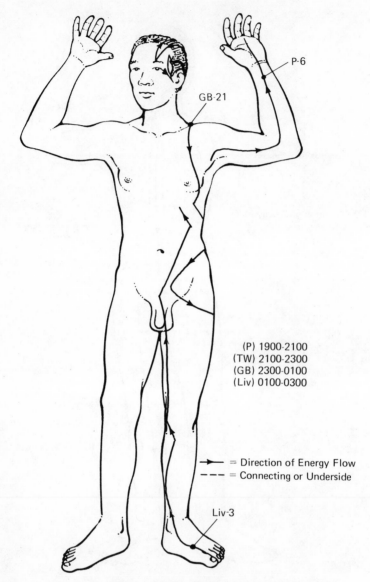

P-6

GB-21

(P) 1900-2100
(TW) 2100-2300
(GB) 2300-0100
(Liv) 0100-0300

⟶ = Direction of Energy Flow
--- = Connecting or Underside

Liv-3

Figure 15-5. Third cycle anterior.

kidneys, suprarenal glands, and ovaries can be found on the corresponding side of the back. Conditions affecting the nerves or vessels of either side of the body will cause changes on the corresponding side of the back.

The changes that can be observed visually may be grouped under

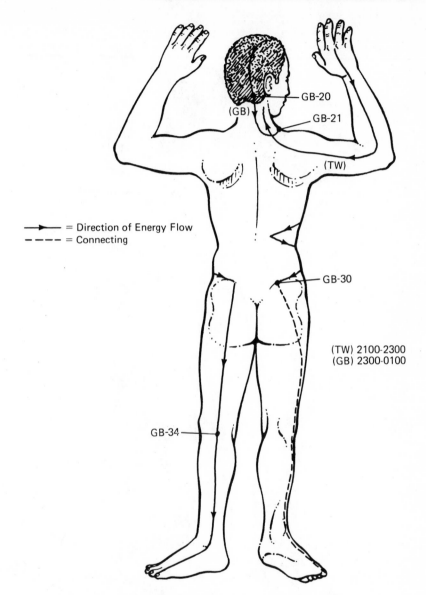

Figure 15-6. Third cycle posterior.

what have for many years been called "trigger points." These include drawn-in bands of tissue, flattened drawn-in areas of tissue, elevated areas giving the impression of localized swelling, atrophy of muscles, hypertrophy of muscles and bony deformities, especially of the spinal column. Many trigger points seem to correlate with acupuncture energy

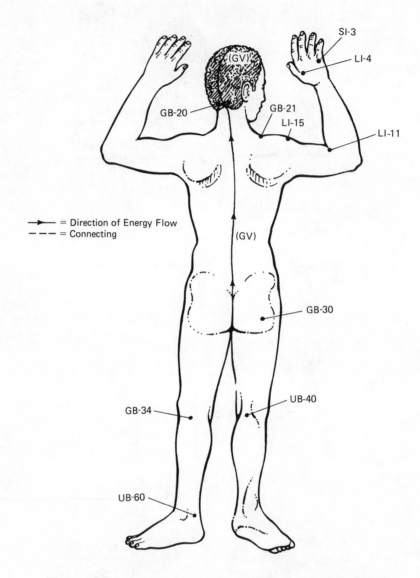

Figure 15-7. Combined posterior points; posterior portion of
GV meridian.

points. According to this theory, pathology in muscles results in tenderness in the muscle, as well as its associated tissues and organs.

It has been evidenced that if the anatomical meridian is cut, the stimulation of an acupuncture point is not transmitted to other points of

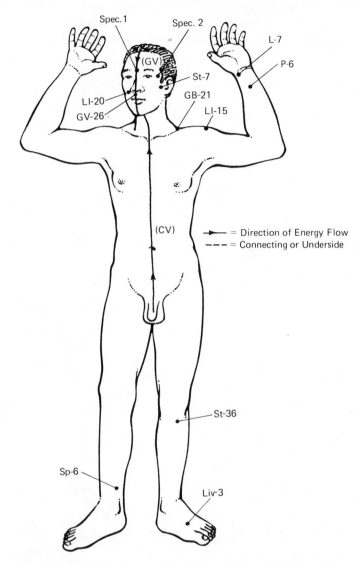

Figure 15-8. Combined anterior points; CV meridian; anterior portion of GV.

the same meridian beyond the level of the cut and the internal organ with which the meridian is associated is not influenced by treatment with acupuncture.[11]

[11] Armstrong, pp. 1582-88.

The word acupuncture combines two Latin words, one being *acus* meaning needle. Therefore, those who use the term acupressure for finger pressure on the acupuncture energy points are in fact saying "needle pressure," which is not at all what they intend to imply. The other word is *punctura*, which means pricking. Therefore, the term acupuncture means needle pricking or the insertion of needles into specific points of the body known as acupuncture points. The following discussion considers how these points can also be effective in massage by applying finger pressure.

TECHNIQUE OF APPLYING FINGER PRESSURE TO ACUPUNCTURE POINTS

When using finger pressure on acupuncture points more than just the amount of pressure applied should be considered. As with all massage, the degree of pressure must be judged in relation to the tolerance of the patient. For this particular technique the more pressure the patient can tolerate, the greater the effectiveness of the treatment. However, judgment must be exercised when dealing with acute pain, swelling, local injuries to the area being treated, and systemic complications. Deeper pressure will probably be needed if the complications are chronic.

Use one finger, usually the middle finger or the thumb, to press against the acupuncture point. Small friction-like circular movements may be used to work one's way toward deeper pressure with the ultimate objective being that of deep, constant pressure on the accurate acupuncture point. Effective treatment time ranges from one to five minutes per point per treatment, or until the patient claims relief. The author has actually heard patients say, in reference to pain, "It's going away . . . It's going away . . . It's gone!"

Some contraindications exist, especially for people who are not fully trained in acupuncture. Avoid using these techniques directly over contusions, scar tissue or infection, or if the patient has a serious cardiac condition. Discontinue treatment immediately if the patient appears aggravated or if no improvement is observable. Children under seven years of age should not be treated with these techniques.

The 20 most useful acupuncture points will be used as examples to indicate the wide variety of disabilities that can be treated effectively using finger pressure to acupuncture points. Pressure application must be applied to the *exact point* or treatment will be useless.

Figure 15-9 and Table 15-2 provide an explanation of proportional cun units, based on the patient's hand measurement, not the acupunc-

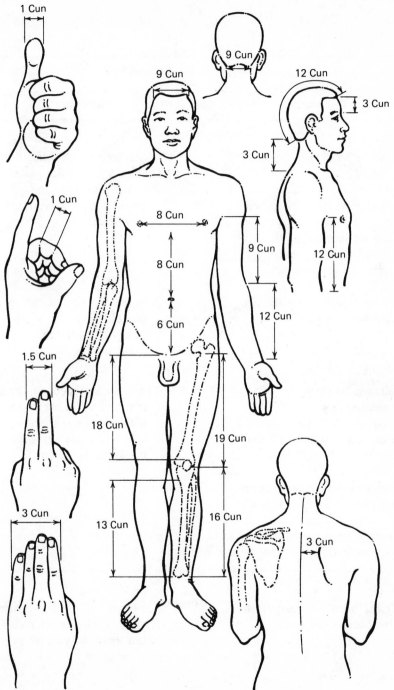

Figure 15-9. Proportional cun units.

Table 15-2

Table for Proportional Measurement

DISTANCE	CUN	REMARKS
Head		
Anterior hairline to posterior hairline	12	If hairlines are indistinguishable, measure the glabella to the process of the seventh cervical vertebra as 18 cun.
Anterior hairline to glabella	3	
Posterior hairline to the process of the seventh cervical vertebra	3	
The hairline between the two temporal regions	9	Between the tips of the two mastoid processes is also measured as 9 cun.
Thorax & Abdomen		
Distance between the two nipples	8	The anterior aspect of chest is measured in accordance with intercostal space. Width of every rib is measured as 1.6 cun.
From lower end of sternum to center of umbilicus	8	
Center of umbilicus to upper border of symphysis pubis	5	
Axillary crease to tip of eleventh rib	12	
Back		
Medial border of scapula to midline of back	3	To locate points lengthwise at the back, the intervertebral space may be taken as a landmark.

Distance	Cun	Remarks
Upper Extremities		
Tranverse axiliary fold to cubital crease	9	Identical for lateral and medial aspects
Cubital crease to transverse wrist crease	12	
Lower Extremities		
Upper level of the greater trochanter to middle of patella	19	Identical for anterior, posterior and lateral aspects.
Middle of patella to tip of lateral malleolus	16	
Upper border of symphysis pubis to upper border of epicondyle of the femur	18	Identical for medial aspect.
Medial condyle of the tibia to the tip of medial malleolus	13	

turist's.[12] Table 15-3 provides information as to the location of these 20 points (see also Figures 15-10 to 15-26 for anatomical diagrams of point locations) and the disabilities indicated that can be partially or totally relieved by pressure at these respective points.

Table 15-4 was compiled by the author using many of the references in the bibliography and with the assistance of Joseph Yao, Donald Courtial, and Dorothy McLaughlin. It is designed to provide quick, easy reference for those using this text to enable them to incorporate finger pressure into their treatment programs.

The idea should be reinforced that any or all of the massage systems described in this text may be used alone or in combination. Any massage system used depends on the responses of individual disabilities and the particular physiological and psychological reactions to the treatment being given, as well as the individual's response to the person providing the treatment.

[12] Reprinted from Academy of Traditional Chinese Medicine, *An Outline of Chinese Acupuncture* (Peking: Foreign Language Press, 1975), pp. 6-7.

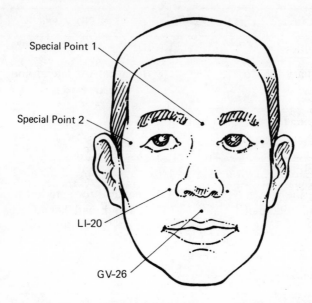

Figure 15-10. Acupuncture points on the face.

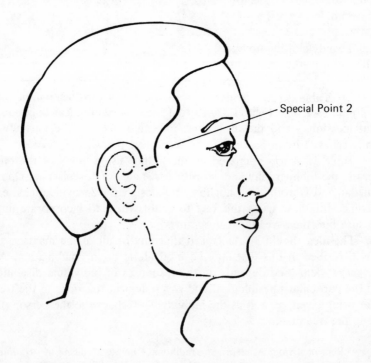

Figure 15-11. Lateral view of Special Point 2 on the face.

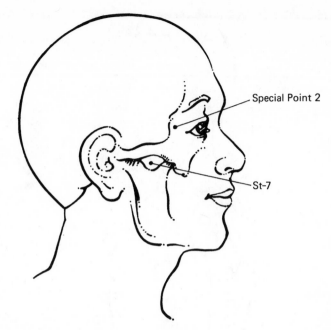

Figure 15-12. Lateral view of Special Points 2 and St. 7 on the face.

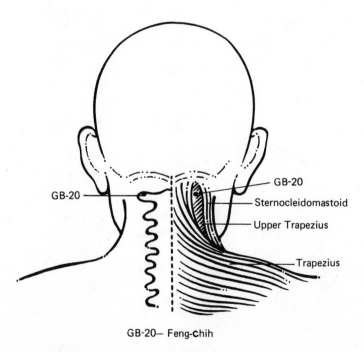

GB-20— Feng-chih

Figure 15-13. Acupuncture point GB-20 Feng-chih.

113

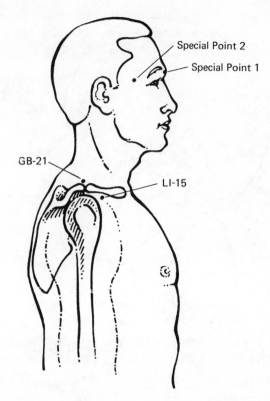

Figure 15-14. Acupuncture point GB-21, Chien-ching, and LI-15 Chien-yu, lateral view.

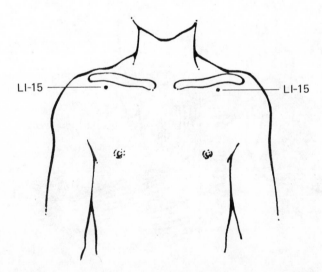

Figure 15-15. Acupuncture point LI-15 Chien-yu, frontal view.

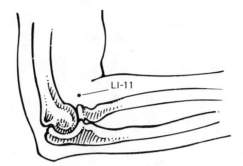

Figure 15-16.   Acupuncture point LI-11 Chu-chih.

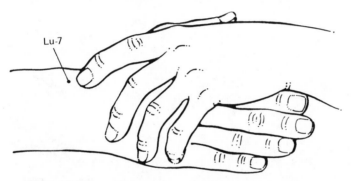

Figure 15-17.   Acupuncture point LU-7 Lieh-chueh.

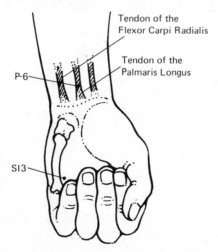

Figure 15-18.   Acupuncture point P-6 Nei-Kuan and S-13 Hou-chi.

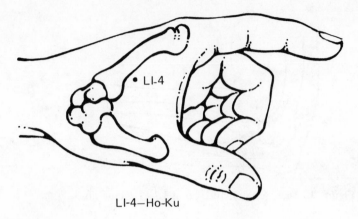

LI-4—Ho-Ku

Figure 15-19. Acupuncture point LI-4 Ho-Ku.

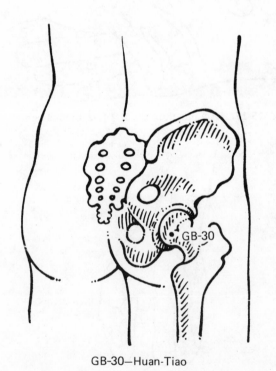

GB-30—Huan-Tiao

Figure 15-20. Acupuncture point GB-30 Huan-tiao, lateral view.

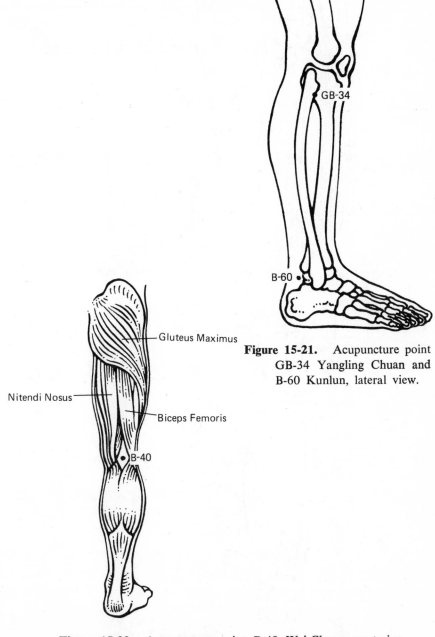

GB-34

B-60

Figure 15-21. Acupuncture point GB-34 Yangling Chuan and B-60 Kunlun, lateral view.

Gluteus Maximus

Nitendi Nosus

Biceps Femoris

B-40

Figure 15-22. Acupuncture point B-40 Wei-Chung, posterior view.

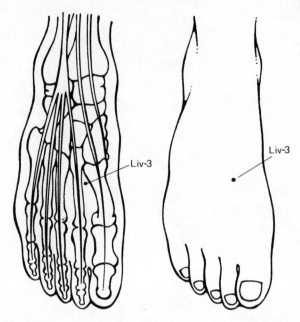

Figure 15-23. Acupuncture point Liv-3 Tai-chung, frontal foot view.

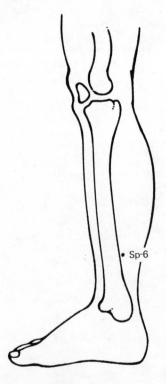

Figure 15-24. Acupuncture point SP-6 San-yin-chiao, lateral view.

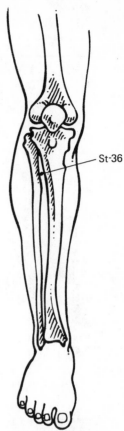

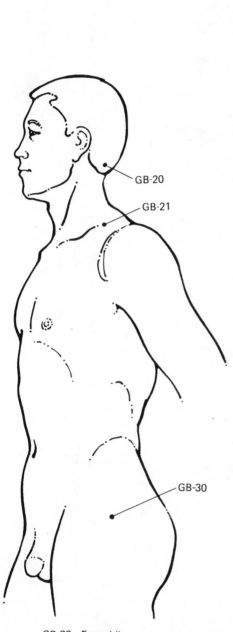

Figure 15-25. Acupuncture point St.-36 Tsu-san-li, frontal view.

GB-20— Feng-chih
GB-21—Chien-ching
GB-30—Huan-tiao

Figure 15-26. Laterial view GB-20 Feng-chih, GB-21 Chien-ching, GB-30 Huan-tiao.

Table 15-3

Location of 20 Most Useful Acupuncture Points

Acupuncture Point	Chinese Name and Meaning	Location	Indications
Urinary Bladder-40 B-40	Wei-Chung "Commanding Middle"	At the center of the popliteal fossa	Low back pain Sciatica Lower extremity paralysis Leg cramp Disorders of hip joint and surrounding soft tissue Knee joint pain, arthritis Heat stroke Apoplexy Epilepsy Acute gastroenteritis Cystitis
Urinary Bladder-60 B-60	Kunlun "Mountain"	Midpoint between the posterior margin of the lateral malleolus and the Achilles tendon	Lower extremity paralysis Low back pain Sciatica Disorders of the ankle joint and surrounding soft tissue

Gall Bladder-20 GB-20	Feng-chih "Wind Pond"	Midpoint of a line joining the tip of the mastoid process to the posterior midline in the groove between the trapezius and the sternocleido-mastoid	Tension headache Migraine headache Stiff neck Dizziness Vertigo Common cold Hypertension Tinnitus
Gall Bladder-21 GB-21	Chieng-ching "Shoulder Well'	Midway between C_7 and acromion process	Shoulder and back pain Neck pain and rigidity Upper extremity motor impairment Mastisis Hyperthyroidism Functional uterine bleeding
Gall Bladder-30 GB-30	Huan-tiao "Jumping Circle"	One-third of the distance from the greater trochanter to the base of the coccyx	Hip joint pain Sciatica Low back pain Lower extremity paralysis Disorders of hip joint and surrounding soft tissue

Table 15-3 Continued

ACUPUNCTURE POINT	CHINESE NAME AND MEANING	LOCATION	INDICATIONS
Gall Bladder-34 GB-34	Yangling Chuan "Yang Mound Spring"	Anterior to the neck of the fibula	Hemiplegia Diseases of the gallbladder Low back pain Dizziness Vertigo Acid regurgitation Lower extremity and knee pain
Governing Vessel-26 GV-26	Jan-chung "Middle of the Man"	One-third of the distance from the inferior surface of the nose to the upper lip line	Shock Heat stroke Low back pain Epilepsy Facial paralysis
Large Intestines-4 LI-4	Ho-Ku "Meeting Valley"	Between first and second metacarpals	Foreheadache Toothache Temporomandibular joint arthritis Tonsilitis Rhinitis

ACUPUNCTURE POINT	CHINESE NAME AND MEANING	LOCATION	INDICATIONS
			Oropharyngitis
			Facial paralysis
			Pain and paralysis of upper extremity
			Hyperhydrosis
			Goiter
			Eye Disease
			Fever
			Hemiplegia
			Analgesic
			Abdominal pain
			Common cold—coughing
			Amenorrhea
			Delirium
			Induction of labor
			Insomnia
			Prostration
			Asthma
			Anesthesia for dental work—especially for lower jaw

Table 15-3   Continued

ACUPUNCTURE POINT	CHINESE NAME AND MEANING	LOCATION	INDICATIONS
Large Intestines-11 LI-11	Chu-chih "Crooked Pond"	Radial end of fold of fully flexed elbow	Shoulder and elbow pain Paralysis of upper extremity Hypertension Disorders of elbow joint and surrounding soft tissue Fever Common cold Chorea Eczema Neurodermatitis
Large Intestines-15 LI-15	Chien-yu "Shoulder Bone"	In the depression of the acromion in the center of the deltoid muscle when the arm is abducted to 90°	Pain and impaired movement of elbow and arm Disorders of shoulder joint and surrounding soft tissue
Large Intestines-20 LI-20	Ying-hsiang "Welcome Fragrance"	At the lower margin and lateral to the nostrils in the nasolabial fold	Facial paralysis Rhinitis Sinusitis Ascariasis of bile duct

Point	Location	Indications
Liver-3 Liv-3 Tai-chung "Too Rushy"	Between the first and second metatarsals, in a fossa, just distal to the heads	Headache Dizziness Epilepsy
Lung-7 Lu-7 Lieh-chueh "Listing Deficiency"	Proximal to styloid process of radius	Headache Neck pain Cough Asthma Facial paralysis
Pericardium-6 P-6 Nei-Kuan "Inner Gate"	Two cun above ventral wrist fold between the tendons of palmaris longus and the flexor carpi radialis	Vomiting Gastralgia Palpitation Angina pectoris Hiccough Chest and costal region pain Stomach pain Insomnia Epilepsy Hysteria

Table 15-3 Continued

ACUPUNCTURE POINT	CHINESE NAME AND MEANING	LOCATION	INDICATIONS
Small Intestines-3 SI-3	Hou-chi "Back Stream"	At the apex of the distal palmar crease on the ulnar side of a clenched fist	Neck pain and rigidity Low back pain Tinnitus Deafness Occipital headache Upper extremity paralysis Night sweating Epilepsy Malaria
Spleen-6 Sp-6	San-yin-chiao "Three Ying Crossing"	Three cun above medial malleolus, just behind the posterior edge of the tibia	Insomnia Barborymus Abdominal distention Loose stool Irregular menstruation Nocturnal emission Impotence Spermatorrhea Orchitis Enuresis Neurasthenia Frequent urination Hemiplegia Urine retention

Stomach-7 St-7	Hsia-Kuan "Lower Gate"	In the depression at the lower border of the zygomatic arch, anterior to the condyloid process of the mandible	Toothache Facial paralysis Trigeminal neuralgia Temporomandibular joint arthritis
Stomach-36 St-36	Tsu-san-li "Walk Three More Miles"	One cun distal and lateral to the tibial tuberosity	Acute and chronic gastritis Nausea and vomiting Functional gastrointestinal disturbances Digestive tract diseases Neurosis Some allergies Fever Shock Aching of hips and knees Leg edema or ache Hemiplegia Anemia Headache Epilepsy Lumbago

Table 15-3 Continued

ACUPUNCTURE POINT	CHINESE NAME AND MEANING	LOCATION	INDICATIONS
			Heaviness of head and frontal headache Acute and chronic enteritis Acute pancreatitis Pyloric spasm Jaundice Urogenital ailments General weakness Paralytic illness
Special Point #1	Yin-tang "Seal Palace"	At the glabella, midway between the medial margins of the eyebrows	Diseases of the nose Headache Dizziness Vertigo
Special Point #2	Tai-yang "Supreme Yang"	At the temple, one cun directly posterior to the midpoint of a line joining the lateral canthus of the eye and the lateral margin of the eyebrow	Migraine Trigeminal neuralgia Eye diseases Toothache Facial paralysis

Table 15-4

Some Combinations of These 20 Points
for Various Disorders

HEADACHE

Frontal—"Heaviness of Head"
Large Intestine 4
Special Point #1
Stomach 36

Vertical Headache
Urinary Bladder 60

Tension Headache
Gall Bladder 20
Gall Bladder 21
Large Intestine 4
Liver 3
Special Point #1

Migraine Headache
Gall Bladder 20
Gall Bladder 36
Large Intestine 4
Liver 3
Special Point #2
Stomach 36

Sinus Headache—Chronic Rhinitis
Gall Bladder 20
Large Intestine 4
Large Intestine 20
Lung 7
Special Point #1

Temporomandibular Headache
Gall Bladder 20
Special Point #2

Occipital Headache
Gall Bladder 20
Gall Bladder 21
Liver 3
Small Intestine 3
Urinary Bladder 60

Trigeminal Nerve—Facial
Paralysis
Governing Vessel 26
Large Intestine 4
Large Intestine 20
Lung 7
Special Point #2
Stomach 7

Generalized Headache
Large Intestine 4
Special Point #1

From Malfunction of the Liver
Large Intestine 4
Large Intestine 11
Urinary Bladder 40

Diseases of the Head, Face, Trunk, and Internal Organs

Gall Bladder 34
Large Intestine 4

Small Intestine 3
Stomach 36

Neck Disorders
Gall Bladder 20
Gall Bladder 21
Lung 7

Table 15-4 Continued

DISORDERS OF THE UPPER EXTREMITY

Shoulder Disorders
 Gall Bladder 21
 Large Intestine 11

Elbow Disorders
 Gall Bladder 21
 Large Intestine 4
 Large Intestine 11
 Large Intestine 15
 Small Intestine 3

DISORDERS OF THE TRUNK AND LOWER EXTREMITY

Low Back Pain
 Gall Bladder 34
 Governing Vessel 34
 Small Intestine 3
 Urinary Bladder 40
 Urinary Bladder 60

Lower Extremity Involvement
Pain, Paralysis, Fatigue
 Gall Bladder 30
 Gall Bladder 34
 Stomach 36
 Urinary Bladder 40
 Urinary Bladder 60

*Disorders of Hip Joint and
Surrounding Soft Tissue*
 Gall Bladder 30
 Gall Bladder 34
 Urinary Bladder 40

Sciatica
 Gall Bladder 30
 Gall Bladder 34
 Urinary Bladder 40
 Urinary Bladder 60

Knee Pain
 Gall Bladder 34
 Large Intestine 4
 Stomach 36
 Spleen 6
 Urinary Bladder 40

*Disorders of the Ankle Joint and
Surrounding Soft Tissue*
 Gall Bladder 34
 Urinary Bladder 60

Muscular Dysfunction of the Feet
 Spleen 6
 Stomach 36

SYSTEMIC DISORDERS

Common Cold
 Gall Bladder 20
 Large Intestine 4
 Large Intestine 20
 Lung 7
 Special Point #1

Impotence
 Stomach 36
 Spleen 6

Insomnia
 Pericardium 6
 Spleen 6

Table 15-4 Continued

Cough
  Lung 7
  Spleen 6
	Irregular Menses
	  Gall Bladder 21
	  Large Intestine 4
	  Spleen 6
	  Stomach 36

Dizziness
  Gall Bladder 20
  Gall Bladder 34
  Liver 3
  Special Point #1
	Morning Sickness
	  Pericardium 6
	  Stomach 36

Epilepsy
  Gall Bladder 34
  Small Intestine 3
	Nausea
	  Pericardium 6
	  Stomach 36

Fever
  Large Intestine 4
  Large Intestine 11
	Shock
	  Pericardium 6
	  Stomach 36

Heat Stroke
  Governing Vessel 26
  Urinary Bladder 40
	Tinnitus
	  Gall Bladder 20
	  Small Intestine 3

Hemiplegia
  Gall Bladder 34
  Large Intestine 4
  Spleen 6
	Toothache
	  Large Intestine 4
	  Large Intestine 20
	  Lung 7
	  Special Point #2
	  Stomach 7

Hypertension
  Gall Bladder 20
  Large Intestine 4
  Large Intestine 11
  Stomach 36
  Spleen 6
	Vertigo
	  Gall Bladder 20
	  Gall Bladder 34
	  Special Point #1

SUMMARY

Since 1958, Western medicine's interest in the effectiveness of acupuncture has increased. Both Eastern and Western medicine are actively involved in research to explain physiologically or psychologically how acupuncture accomplishes anesthesia and even euphoria. The reasons for

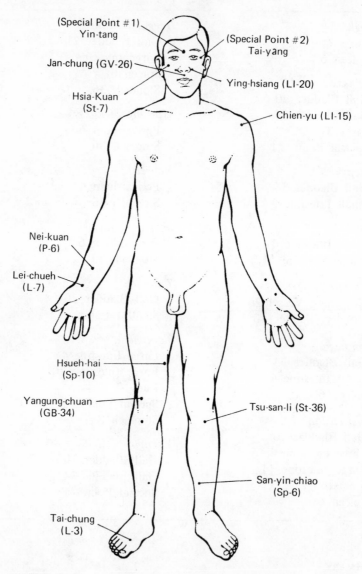

(Special Point #1)
Yin-tang

(Special Point #2)
Tai-yang

Jan-chung (GV-26)

Hsia-Kuan
(St-7)

Ying-hsiang (LI-20)

Chien-yu (LI-15)

Nei-kuan
(P-6)

Lei-chueh
(L-7)

Hsueh-hai
(Sp-10)

Yangung-chuan
(GB-34)

Tsu-san-li (St-36)

San-yin-chiao
(Sp-6)

Tai-chung
(L-3)

Figure 15-27. Total body frontal view of acupuncture points.

its effectiveness become clearer as research continues in the methods of pain relief and endorphins (endogenous morphine, Chapter 6).

This section has presented a brief history of acupuncture as well as a discussion of the Oriental theories related to meridians. The discussion of 20 selected points provides the reader with general knowledge of the

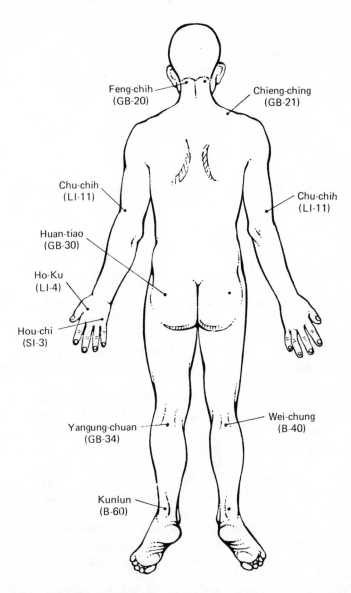

Figure 15-28. Total body posterior view of acupuncture points.

most commonly used points and the disabilities that can effectively benefit from finger pressure on specific points. The bibliography provides
complete information related to hundreds of other acupuncture points.
The reader should pursue the literature for more complete information.

Chapter 16

Shiatsu

In Japanese *shi* means "fingers." *Atsu* means "pressure." Thus, *Shiatsu* literally means treating the body with applied finger pressure. Application depends on the instinct of the individual who treats himself—applying pressure at the point of discomfort—or the expertise of the one giving the treatment, who can find sensitive areas with skilled hands.

The thumbs and palms of the hands are used to apply pressure to certain points to maintain or improve health, and contribute to the cure of certain illnesses. In treating the face and abdomen, use the index, middle and ring fingers. The palm of the hand is used to apply pressure to the eyes and abdomen when applying vibration.

Pressure should be firm, using the soft bulbs of the fingers or thumbs. Pressure should be gentle and perpendicular to the area being treated. To treat a specific disability, points nearest the disability are usually used. Sometimes, however, pressure on distant areas is believed to bring improvement. (Example: Pressure on the sole of the foot for kidney disease or on the left hand to affect problems of the heart may be applied.)

Duration of a single application of Shiatsu pressure should be from five to seven seconds. It should cause a sensation midway between pleasure and pain. (Many patients will say, "It hurts good.") Each area can be treated in about three minutes. Total treatment should never last more than an hour, and a normal treatment would be approximately 30 minutes.

In his book on *Shiatsu*, Tokujiro Namikoshi uses many points that are similar to acupuncture points.[1] (For location of acupuncture points, refer to Chapter 15.) The acupuncture point for relief of weariness, for example, is St.-36. Namikoshi's shiatsu interpretation claims this area as a "sanri" point or "three ri" (literally, 7.5 miles). Both interpretations imply relief for weary walkers. See Figure 15-23.

In a more recent book, however, Wataru Ohashi accurately follows the ancient acupuncture points working with the meridians, replacing needles with finger pressure.[2] Ohashi advocates the practice of Shiatsu within the family circle as a means of achieving better communication, lessening family conflict, and promoting happiness, health, and love.

[1] Tokujiro Namikoshi, *Shiatsu, Health and Vitality at Your Fingertips* (San Francisco, Calif.: Japan Publications, Inc., 1969), p. 22.

[2] Wataru Ohashi, *Do It Yourself Shiatsu* (Toronto: Clark Irwin & Co., Ltd., 1976). For a complete discussion of his method, refer to his text.

Chapter 17

The Bindegewebsmassage System

GENERAL PRINCIPLES

Both Eastern and Western medical philosophies assume that isolated pathologies do not exist anywhere in the human body. The entire organism functions as a balanced and coordinated unit if the body is healthy. Any disability that disrupts this harmony affects the autonomic and central nervous system as well as hormonal and humoral systems. In all cases the body must be considered as a physiological and psychological whole.

PHYSIOLOGY OF BINDEGEWEBSMASSAGE

The most superficial layer of the tissues forming the body surface is the skin. It is the immediate link with the external environment. It contains the exteroceptors, i.e., specialized nerve endings which react to touch in various intensities and to changes in temperature such as heat and cold.

The material presented in this chapter reflects the viewpoint of the Elisabeth Dicke School in Uberlingen, West Germany, where the author of this book studied. In addition to Dicke's *Meine Bindegewebsmassage* (Hippokrates-Verlag, Stuttgart, 1956), Marie Ebner's book, *Connective Tissue Massage* (The Williams and Wilkins Co., Baltimore, Md., 1962) was very helpful since it clarified many points which were difficult to understand in Dicke's text. However, the material in this chapter is Dicke's Bindegewebsmassage as the author learned it in Uberlingen and it varies from Ebner's text in many ways.

The deepest layer forming the body surface is that of the muscles. These too contain numerous nerve endings that can alter the tension in the tissue both reflexively and voluntarily. These nerve endings also register alterations in the tension of the tissue by means of proprioceptors, i.e., specialized nerve endings sensitive to alterations in the length of the muscle fiber. Both these tissues relate to the somatic and the autonomic nervous systems. Therefore, vascular changes occur in both tissues.

The layer of tissue between skin and muscle consists of connective tissue, and this is the layer of tissue that is thought to be particularly important when applying Bindegewebsmassage.

It is considered that organic disturbances follow vascular channels over arterial reflexes. It is believed that these reactions are responsible for many pathological disturbances which cannot be explained as reflex symptoms within the segmental distribution. The Bindegewebsmassage system of massage is based on the concept that these reactions are responsible for certain disabilities. This may explain why some cases claim removal of peripheral symptoms through massage of the connective tissue to the back. These segments do not correspond to the dermatome area in the periphery. (See Figure 17-1 for the back areas which correspond to visceral pathologies as described by MacKenzie.) This information is taken largely from German sources, but the beneficial effect of the treatment has been confirmed by the experiences of people of many nationalities.

At the beginning of a treatment program one should proceed cautiously to build up tolerance to these procedures. Begin with the basic strokes, the Grundaufbau. Then, if the patient tolerates it well, one can proceed to the thoracic and cervical segments. To proceed faster, to treat, or even to demonstrate the strokes out of sequence will bring about undesired reflex effects which will only frighten the patient and delay progress.[1] While one must begin treatment carefully, one should also terminate all treatment with the basic and balancing strokes within the area treated.

Dicke lists and defines exact strokes and systematic treatment for various individual circumstances. Ebner also uses the case method approach, demonstrating the exact injury or disability and complete information which accompanies each case. This includes the patient's sex, age, and occupation, as well as Ebner's own examination and evaluation, and the patient's description of symptoms. A record of that which can be seen and felt, range of motion, pain, swelling in specific

---

[1] The author has found this to be true by experience.

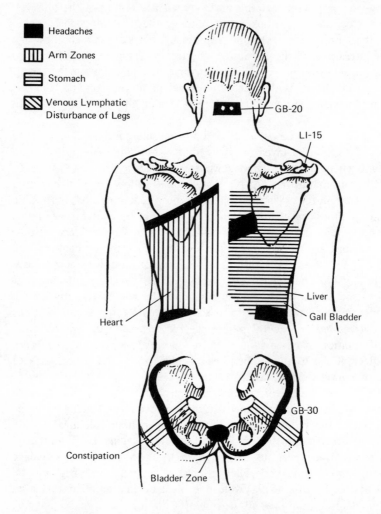

Headaches
Arm Zones
Stomach
Venous Lymphatic
Disturbance of Legs

GB-20

LI-15

Liver

Heart

Gall Bladder

Constipation

GB-30

Bladder Zone

Figure 17-1. Some connective tissue zones and acupuncture
points on the back.

anatomical areas and treatment given, with exact notes of progress for
each treatment is also included. Ebner, in certain instances, starts with
the basic section and on the same day proceeds directly to the involved
anatomical area of disability, unlike Dicke's strict adherence to the
total system.

By studying Figure 17-1 one can see the areas of the back that
Bindegewebsmassage relates to visceral problems, headache, etc. Begin
with the basic strokes to the level of the disorder before concentrating

the strokes. Deviations from normal can be felt by the fingers, including tension, localized swelling, depressed areas, drawn-in bands of tissue, atrophy of muscles or hypertrophy of muscles. Extreme tenderness in any involved area requires a very gentle approach leading gradually toward deeper pressure according to the patient's tolerance.

The patient should have no discomfort upon termination of the massage. Balancing strokes, and strokes treating the great trochanter or subcostal areas should return natural and comfortable sensations to the patient.

Dicke presents numerous disabilities that respond to this massage system, all of which are treated by the strokes described and illustrated here which follow segmental distribution upward on the spinal column to the level of enervation. Two main types of pathologies respond especially well: changes in peripheral structures due to interference with their blood supply; and changes in peripheral structures which have occurred due to pathological conditions related to other parts of the segmental distribution.

Dicke lists the following specific disabilities which respond well with Bindegewebsmassage treatment:

Skin and Under-Skin—symmetrical eczema, ichthyosis, itching skin, neurodermatitis, phlegmon, decubitus, scars.

Bones and Joints—fractures, orthopedic cases, periarthritis, epicondylitis, tendo-vaginitis, arthritis, arthrosis.

Musculature—myalgia, lumbago, torticollis, progressive muscular dystrophy.

Nerves—after treatment of neuritis, neuralgia, ischialgia, brachial neuralgia.

Blood and Lymph Vessels—varicose symptoms complex, thrombophlebitis (subacute), hemorrhoids, edema.

Circulatory Disturbances—"Raynaud's" disease, Burger's disease, intermittent claudication, arteriosclerotic and diabetic gangrene, scleroderma, frostbite, trophic disturbances, Sudeck's atrophy.

Inner Organs

Heart and Circulatory Diseases—hypertonia, angina pectoris, myocardial dysfunctions, infarcts (subacute), functional disturbances.

Respiratory Diseases—bronchial asthma, chronic bronchitis, bronchiectasis, emphysema, post-operative situations.

Stomach Diseases—acute and chronic gastritis, ulcers, gastric atony, cardiospasms, functional disturbances.

Intestinal Diseases—spastic and atonic constipation, chronic colitis, colica mucosa, post-op appendectomy.

Liver-Gall Bladder System Diseases—hepatitis (subacute), cholesystitis (subacute), post-op gall bladder and bile duct operations.

Diseases of the Kidneys and Urinary Systems—nephritis and pyelitis postoperative and subacute conditions, enuresis nocturna.

Gynecological Diseases—infection of the ovaries and uterus (subacute and postoperative conditions).

Endocrine Disturbances—amenorrhea, dysmenorrhea, lactation, genital infantilism, hyperthyroidism.

Central Nervous System Diseases—after treatment of poliomyelitis, encephalitis, "Little's" disease, multiple sclerosis, Parkinson's disease.

Various Headaches—posttraumatic and rheumatic headache, migraines.

Sense Organ Diseases—nose (cold), ears, eyes.

Allergies—hay fever, bronchial asthma, eczema (of skin).

Contraindications

Tuberculosis at all stages, all malignant tumors, myoma and endometriosis; psychosis and mental illnesses.

HISTORY OF BINDEGEWEBSMASSAGE

Bindegewebsmassage was developed by Elisabeth Dicke of Germany, who, in 1929, suffered from a severe disturbance in the peripheral circulation of her right leg. As a result of a neglected tooth infection, a general toxemia developed, which resulted in an endarteritis obliterans of the right leg. This leg was cold and bluish in color, the toes giving the appearance of incipient gangrene. The dorsalis pedis artery was no longer palpable. Frau Dicke was advised to consider amputation of the lower limb.

In addition to the extreme pain in the extremity, she suffered from an almost unbearable backache. While lying on her side she tried to give herself some relief by massaging over the painful areas of her back. She found that over the sacrum and the right iliac crest, thickenings and infiltrations could be palpated, while toward the left side on the same level, the skin felt tight.

She tried to ease the tension by massage with her fingers across the affected areas, but found that these areas were hypersensitive to touch. Slight stroking with the fingertip caused great pain. The tension, however, gradually subsided, the pain in the back eased, and an agreeable sensation of warmth took its place. On successive days she persisted with the stroking which was done by other people. She gradually felt pins and needles in the affected leg, followed by a sensation of warmth.

In further treatments she incorporated the areas around the greater trochanter and along the iliotibial tract. Gradually the superficial venous circulation reappeared in the thigh and leg. The severe symptoms subsided after three more months of treatment carried out by a colleague under Frau Dicke's direction. She was able to resume her occupation after a year.

Years of investigation followed. During the course of her illness Frau Dicke had experienced pathological function of internal organs in addition to the symptoms in the back and leg. She suffered from a chronic gastritis, the liver showed enlargement, the heart showed symptoms of angina, and finally she experienced disturbance of kidney function. These visceral complaints cleared up simultaneously with the improvement of peripheral circulation and normalization of tissue changes in the back. Treatment of pathologically affected areas of the body surface helped to clear up pathological changes in affected viscera. She discovered that certain areas on the body surface definitely related to certain viscera.

Systemic observation of patients in the following years confirmed these findings. Unknown to Dicke at the time, the English neurologist Head had already described similar findings, showing changes in the same well-defined areas of the body surface, pertaining to specific organs. These alterations appear when pathological changes take place in affected viscera. These are known in the literature as "Head Zones" (see Chapter 15). The ancient Chinese, of course, became aware thousands of years ago of an increased sensitivity of certain skin areas (called points) when a body organ or function was impaired.[2]

"Further clinical investigations followed in 1935 under Professor Veil in Jena and in 1938 under Professor Kohlrausch and Dr. Tierich H. Leube in Freiburg, incorporating the basic work of J. MacKenzie. While Head pointed out changes in skin areas, MacKenzie (1917)

[2] See discussion of the history of acupuncture, Chapter 15.

drew attention to changes in muscle tone and sensitivity in areas which share the same root supply with pathologically affected organs." [3]

Years of work and investigation resulted in the present-day method of Bindegewebsmassage in Germany. This method is now used in many other countries, being widely employed not only in pathological conditions associated with visceral disease, but also in the treatment of diseases associated with the pathology of circulation. In this it shows very gratifyng results. In Germany, it is also widely used by members of the medical profession for diagnostic purposes.

POSITION OF THE PATIENT

The patient may be in a sitting position for treatment; the patient may also be treated in a prone-lying or side-lying position.

POSITION OF THE ONE GIVING THE MASSAGE

As with other massage techniques, the operator should be in any position, be it seated or standing, which provides for good body mechanics and avoids fatigue.

APPLICATION OF TECHNIQUE

Using the pad of the middle finger, touch the patient's skin very firmly without applying more pressure than is necessary. Fingernails must be very short. The strokes must be applied with even pressure and speed.

GENERAL PRINCIPLES OF BINDEGEWEBSMASSAGE

Each stroke is done three times. The right side is done first, then the left side. Loss of hand contact occurs with completion of each stroke. The hand which is not working is kept in touch with the patient at all times. Use the third fingertip and let the fourth finger follow. Get your pull through the entire arm. Feel for spinal and pelvic bony structures and follow their edges. *Use no lubricant.*

Flat strokes are done by using more "finger area" and a lighter stroke. Steep strokes are done with less finger area and deeper pressure. Exploration of the body tissues will reveal tightness in certain areas, as well as flattened or drawn areas. The fingers applying pressure will often "skip" when they encounter such areas. Localized swelling can

[3] Ebner, p. 3.

be felt. Atrophy or hypertrophy of muscles can be noticed. Even bony deformities can at times be felt. Mobility of the layers of connective tissue can be evaluated. Painful areas can be assessed. Palpation of the muscles will give information as to the degree of tension present. Any asymmetry or muscle imbalance can be felt.

Grip the tissues between the thumb and fingers, lifting them away from the superficial layer. In some areas it may be impossible to lift the tissues if they are tight and/or painful. This usually indicates a pathological condition. See Figure 17-1 for reflex areas on the back that relate to visceral pathologies as discovered by Head and MacKenzie. There are also areas on the back that relate to headache, constipation, arterial diseases of the legs, and venous lymphatic disorders of the legs. Drawn-in areas over the scapula and posterior deltoid indicate disorders of the upper extremity.

By pulling from the fifth lumbar vertebrae to the occiput, first on one side of the spine, then on the other, abnormal areas will become red or even raise a wheal. The spinal level can indicate areas of involvement. This is called the diagnostic stroke. Care must be taken that the pressure of this stroke is not painfully deep. The third finger leads and the fourth finger follows. The angle of the strokes is between 40 and 60 degrees. *Pull*, do not *push* the tissues under the fingers.

Uncomfortable feelings may be reported by the patient, including a cutting or a scratching sensation, or a feeling of dull pressure. This indicates a pathological condition. If the fingers find it hard to "pull through" tight areas they should not be forced. Depending on body build, age, and other normal conditions of the body, some deviations occur in every normal human being. All findings should be indicated in writing on a chart or diagram. Progress should also be recorded.

Direction of Strokes

In the paravertebral areas the stroke follows the direction of the dermatomes. In the periphery it follows the direction of the muscle fibers, muscle, fascia, tendons, or at right angles to facial borders.

Procedures for Treatment

The back is divided into three sections, the "basic" section, the "thoracic" section, and the "cervical" section. The basic section (*grundaufbau*) includes the coccyx through the first lumbar vertebrae. No treatment is ever given without covering the basic section with a "build up" of the back strokes to the level of the part of the body involved; in cases of the upper extremity all three parts precede local treatment.

Precautions

Adverse effects such as nausea, dizziness, fainting, diarrhea, and profuse perspiration may result if treatment is too harsh or done improperly. The person giving the massage should watch the patient intently; should any of the above become apparent balancing strokes should be done immediately.

BALANCING STROKES

For thoracic balancing strokes the patient should be standing. Stroke with flat, gentle fingers on the right side three times. From T_{12} follow the lower border of the last rib, around the chest, to the mammillary line, pulling very gently, lifting the tissue slightly at the end of the stroke. Repeat this same technique three times on the left.

The five pectoral balancing strokes are as follows: (1) from the middle third of the sternum to the axillary line; (2) from the middle third of the sternum to a little above the end of the first stroke; (3) from the upper third of the sternum to the capsule of the shoulder; (4) from the top of the sternum glide along the lower border of the clavicle; and, (5) out to the capsule of the shoulder. Repeat this technique until the series of five strokes are done three times, first on the right side and then repeated on the left side.

The "great balancing stroke" goes from C_7 to the coccyx. A flat bilateral stroke is done down the erector spinae group to L_5, where the hands separate and follow the line of the rhombus to the posterior inferior spine of the ilium. Then, continue diagonally downward to the

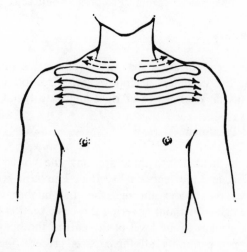

Figure 17-2. Balancing strokes.

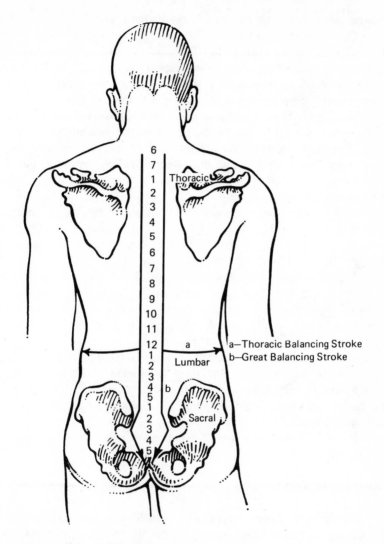

Figure 17-3.   Balancing strokes.

anal fold and coccyx. Repeat this technique three times (see Figures 17-2, 17-3).

THE BASIC TREATMENT (GRUNDAUFBAU)

From Coccyx Through L$_1$

Stroke from the posterior inferior spine of the ilium downward to the coccyx on the right side three times. Repeat on the left. These strokes may be steep unless tension causes pain or other adverse effects.

These strokes are followed by strokes from the posterior inferior spine of the ilium upward to L_5. The stroke ends in a "hook-on"; first on the right side three times, then repeat on the left. A hook-on is frequently used to complete a stroke. The fingers make a comma-shaped, short, deep stroke at the end of a longer stroke.

Next, give three pelvis strokes on the right side. Follow the crest of the ilium, from L_5 around the pelvis to the anterior superior iliac spine. Finish the stroke with a light pulling up of the tissue. Repeat three times. Then, stroke from the posterior inferior spine of the ilium around the pelvis to the anterior superior iliac spine. Finish with a light pulling up of the tissue.

Now, stroke from the anal fold. Stroke behind and under the tuberosity of the ischium around the greater trochanter of the femur and below it, over the tensor fascia lata, then upward in front to the anterior superior iliac spine. Repeat this on the left side.

After this, give a series of hook-ons. Start on the right side and go around with five little hook-ons from L_5 to L_1, the first hook-on L_5 to L_4 beginning on the medial border of the erector spinae, ending at spinous process; continue to L_1. Alternate these strokes right and left until each side has been done three times.

The fan strokes are flat, soft pulls, diagonally downward, in an area between an imaginary line from the highest point on the pelvic crest to the L_3. Each stroke ends in the lumbosacral joint. Alternate the entire fan stroke right and left, until done three times on both sides (see Figure 17-4).

From the basic strokes the system moves upwards along the vertebral column.

From T_{12} to T_7

The person giving the massage should be standing. Administer five hook-on strokes which proceed from T_{12} to T_7, alternating from right to left. Repeat this series three times.

Continue with intercostal strokes, seven gentle ascending strokes beginning over the lowest rib from the posterior border of the anterior axillary line. Each stroke ends with a small hook-on on the vertebrae from T_{12} to T_6.

The seven additional strokes are used only in special treatment for chest conditions. They are the exact reverse of the preceding intercostal strokes.

Pectoral balance strokes, as previously described, are done at this point. Add two strokes which follow the superior border of the

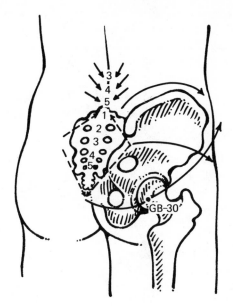

Figure 17-4.   Basic strokes.

clavicle, going from medial to lateral (see Figure 17-2).

The next section of strokes goes from T_7 to C_7. Start and finish on the right. Proceed to the left only if treating both sides. With heart disease do not treat the left side. Usually only one shoulder is treated.

Then, treat the upper extremity in the following steps. Beginning on the right side, do gentle hook-ons from T_7 to C_7 alternating to the left side, three times on each side. Stroke from the vertebral column to the scapula with five strokes beginning from T_7 to the inferior angle of the scapula, working upward and finishing each stroke with a hook-on under the scapula. If swelling is found, do not treat above that level. Pull from the inferior angle of the scapula upward, following *under* the scapula's spinal border to the level of the spine of the scapula three times, using steep strokes. With a "flat" gentle stroke, follow the axillary border of the scapula over the teres major. Be gentle when approaching the axillary region. Stay above the axillary line. With the heel of the hand on the shoulder (with bent fingers) follow the superior aspect of the spine of the scapula from the vertebrae to the axillary aspect of the scapula. This is a pivot-like stroke (see Figure 17-5).

To accomplish widening of the shoulder joint, brace the hypothenar eminence of the hand near the border of the latissimus dorsi. Have fingers reach under the tendon of the latissimus dorsi and pull

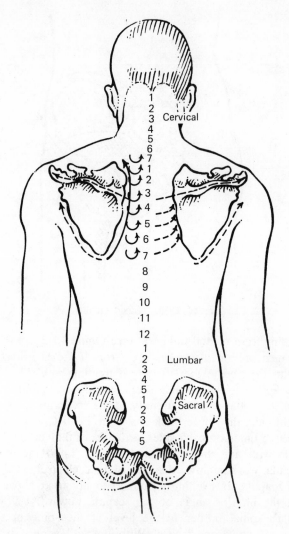

Note: Not All Strokes Are Illustrated Bilaterally.
Follow Written Instructions.

Figure 17-5. Pivot-like strokes.

by flexing the fingers in the palm. While standing and holding the tissues with one hand, stroke the latissimus dorsi *toward* the insertion with a short stroke upward. Stretch the pectorals pulling from the inferior angle of the scapula to the tendon of the pectorals.

Prepare for the next strokes with short, little friction, circular strokes, first on the latissimus tendon, then on the pectorals. Standing at the side of the patient, tuck each hand into one side of the armpit. "Widen" the joint by letting the hands fall open, stretching the pectorals and the latissimus dorsi.

From the inferior angle of the scapula, stroke back toward the scapula to the ventral aspect of the axillary border, stretching the latissimus tendon and stroking over the serratus anterior. Alternate with similar strokes in a reverse direction to stretch the pectorals at the end of the stroke. Crossing the hands, alternately stroke toward the latissimus dorsi, then toward the pectorals. Support the lower trapezius with the left hand and stroke toward the shoulder (see Figures 17-6, 17-7).

The next section goes from C_7 to C_1. The "sun stroke" (see Figure 17-8), in five short strokes which begin on a diagonal, strokes toward C_7. Begin on the lower right side working toward the top right side of C_7.

Ascend from C_7 through C_1 with a light pull along the side of the spinous processes (Figure 17-9). Alternate right to left three times. Administer hook-ons from C_7 to C_1.

Be sure to stabilize the head with the opposing hand alternating right to left three times. Stroke straight across the nuchal line three times in each direction. (Figure 17-9.) (Pectoral balancing may be included, if necessary, on the lower rhombus strokes for balance—Figure 17-2.) Give an ascending small stroke along the anterior upper two-thirds of the right trapezius to its origin. Lightly outline the right sternocleidomastoid, staying on the posterior border from its origin up to its insertion on the mastoid bone (Figure 17-10).

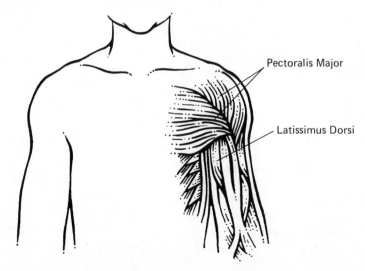

Pectoralis Major

Latissimus Dorsi

Figure 17-6. Widening of the shoulder joint.

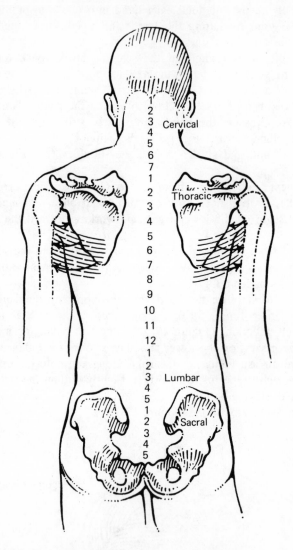

Cervical

Thoracic

Lumbar

Sacral

Note: Not All Strokes Are Illustrated.

Figure 17-7. Widening of the shoulder joint.

Repeat on the left side three times. Using both hands stroke from the anterior trapezius across it. This is a bilateral small stroke, which pulls across the ascending trapezius to just below C_7. This is a balancing stroke (Figures 17-2, 17-3). Use a final balancing stroke from C_7 to the coccyx as previously described.

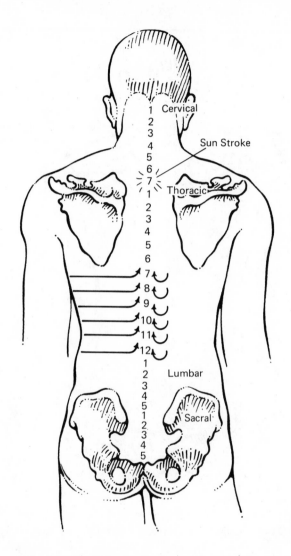

Note: All of the Following Represent "Hook On" Strokes

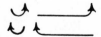

Figure 17-8.   Rib strokes and hook-ons, T_{12} to T_7, sun stroke.

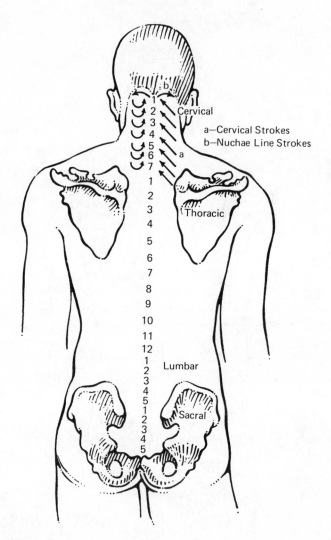

Figure 17-9. Upper back strokes C_7 to C_1.

Treatment for Chest

Asthma may be made worse if this technique is not done exactly right. The person giving the treatment should be standing. Do all the basic strokes followed by the thoracic build-up if the patient will tolerate it. Otherwise, do only the basic strokes until the patient can tolerate the treatment. Add strokes in the reverse direction of the intercostal strokes. Do the right side first, then the left, three times each side, finishing on the right side. Continue with cross strokes from the right to the left and

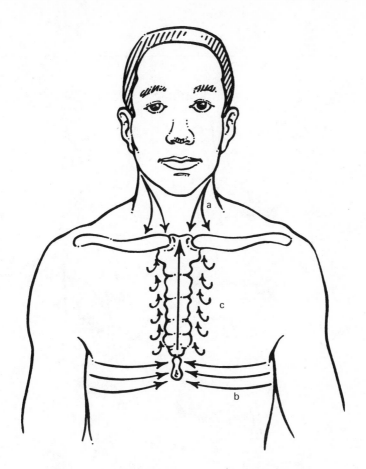

Note: Not All Strokes Are Illustrated; Please Follow the
Written Instructions.

Figure 17-10.   Treatment for the chest, anterior.

left to right between the scapula up to the spine of the scapula (Figure
17-11). Do widening of the shoulder joint (Figures 17-6, 17-7).

Give intercostal strokes toward the sternum from the posterior
axillary line. Give four strokes, repeating the last one in the same place.
Provide a long stroke the length of the sternum from the zyphoid upward
to the interclavicular ligament. Give hook-ons to the sternum, first on
the right and then on the left, alternating sides. Give short, flat strokes
to the sternocleidomastoid insertion. Then use short strokes between the
clavicles over the interclavicular ligament proceeding across the manubrium. Pectoral balance strokes should be included for the benefit of the
patient (Figure 17-2).

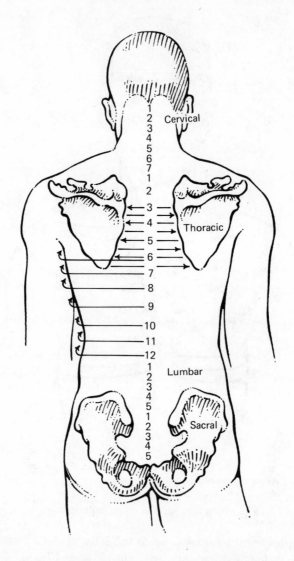

Figure 17-11. Treatment for the chest, posterior.

Strokes across the sternum from its lower end upwards, working across the manubrium, should be administered next. Pectoral strokes are done as a treatment stroke with hook-ons at the end of the stroke (see Figure 17-10). The pectoral stroke is done as a balance stroke. Provide a long stroke from the twelfth rib up to C_7.

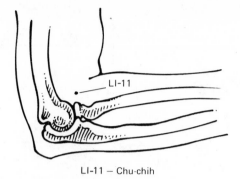

LI-11 — Chu-chih

Figure 17-12.   Elbow and forearm.

Wrist, Hand and Fingers

With the exception of stroking from proximal to distal, Elisabeth Dicke's strokes cover the hand completely. This author prefers most massage strokes to proceed from distal to proximal.

To perform these strokes the operator uses the soft pads of the middle finger, pulling with some depth from proximal to distal. Both thumbs rest on the patient's wrist with no pressure during these strokes.

All strokes previously described can be adapted to these smaller areas and must be mastered.

As illustrated in Figure 17-13a, the first stroke pulls over the lower third of the flexor carpi radialis. The second stroke pulls over the palmaris longus (Figure 17-13b). The third stroke pulls over the flexor carpi ulnaris (Figure 17-13c).

These are followed by short strokes over the volar ligament. Be careful not to press too deeply over the median nerve. Stabilize above the wrist. Get the pull by flexing the fingers. Start on the radial side and work toward the ulnar side (Figure 17-14).

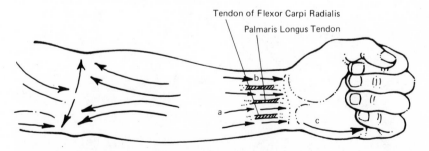

Tendon of Flexor Carpi Radialis
Palmaris Longus Tendon

Figure 17-13.   Elbow and forearm.

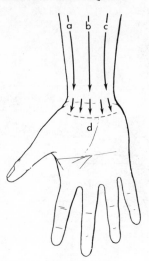

Figure 17-14. Stroking the Palmaris Longus.

Next, follow with short strokes over the transverse ligament across the heel of the hand from thenar to hypothenar eminences (Figure 17-15a). Then long strokes are done over the palmar fascia, working deep to the interossei, pulling toward the fingers (Figure 17-15b). Thenar strokes, which are half ellipsoid, are then given over the inner surface of the thenar eminence (Figure 17-15c).

Transverse strokes are then done over the thenar eminence, working from the inner border outward toward the dorsal surface (Figure

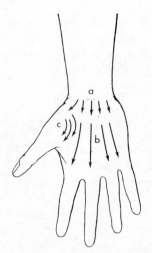

Figure 17-15. Stroking the hand.

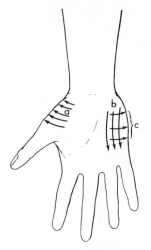

Figure 17-16. Transverse and hypothenar strokes of the hand.

17-16a). Hypothenar strokes of a similar nature are done in a longitudinal direction (Figure 17-16b) and in a transverse direction (Figure 17-16c).

Small, interdigital, longitudinal strokes over the transverse palmaris ligament between the heads of the metacarpals should then be done (Figure 17-17).

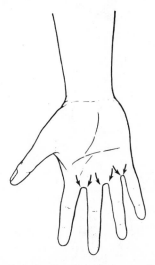

Figure 17-17. Longitudinal strokes over the transverse palmaris ligament.

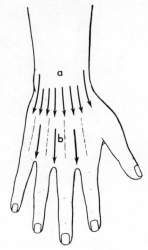

Figure 17-18. Strokes over the transverse palmaris ligament, the interossei, and the dorsum of the hand.

On the dorsum of the hand, short strokes should be done. Anchor the thumb on the volar side. Start radially over the ligamentum dorsalis, and go distally across the ligament adding gentle, passive extension of the wrist simultaneously (Figure 17-18).

Next, perform long, flat gentle strokes over the interossei (Figure 17-18b).

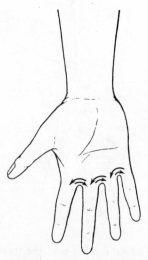

Figure 17-19. Pulling stroke over the fingers.

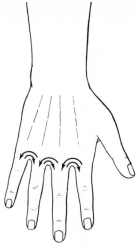

Figure 17-20. Counterpull.

The following stroke is best done with the thumbs. It is a pull and counterpull to stretch the web between the fingers. One hand holds, while the other pulls the next finger away, providing gentle passive motion as well as stroking. Begin on the radial side and work toward the ulnar side. This should be done to both the volar and dorsal surfaces of the hand (Figures 17-19 and 17-20).

Massage of the Fingers

Each finger should be massaged before going on to the next one.

Pull out the long tendons on the volar side of the fingers, stroking the tendon from metacarpophalangeal joint to the tip of the finger. Use one hand to support the patient's hand, to prevent hyperextension of the finger, and to get the proper pressure. *This pulling is not done by grasping the finger, but by stroking along the tendon* (Figure 17-21a). Next, perform small strokes on the medial and lateral borders of the first two phalanges (Figure 17-21b). Follow this by stroking, proximal to distal, with a *little* stretch, over the collateral ligaments of each joint. *Do not pull* into the joint space or go beyond one joint at a time (Figure 17-21c). Stretching of the small joints can be done (Figure 17-21d).

Stretch each joint of each finger by using both thumbs on the dorsal side and both third fingers, pulling outward (Figure 17-22).

Next, apply short strokes over the dorsal aponeurosis, beginning on the thumb. Stretch the long extensor tendons between each joint (Figure 17-23). If the lumbercales are involved, stroke laterally between each joint.

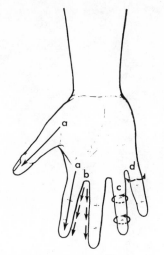

Figure 17-22. Stretching the finger joints.

Figure 17-21. Massage of the fingers.

Stretch the palmar fascia in the following fashion. With the thumbs on the dorsum of the patient's hand, the operator pronates his own hands, stretching the palm of the patient's hand. The volar aspect of the patient's hand is supported by the hypothenar aspect of the operator's hand. Start at the carpal area and work distally with each stroke (Figure 17-24).

Although Dicke would not do so, this author recommends stroking

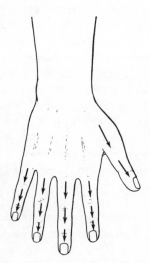

Figure 17-23. Stretching the finger joints.

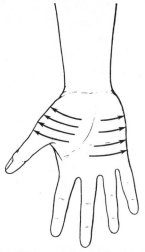

Figure 17-24. Stretching the palmar fascia.

off the entire extremity with effleurage, working from firm pressure gradually toward lighter pressure, and finishing with light effleurage strokes
which follow the venous flow.

Lower Extremity

Precede treatment of the leg with the basic treatment. The patient
is in a seated position if possible. Then ask the patient to lie in a supine
position. Face the patient and always stabilize the patient's leg with the
free hand. As before, all strokes are done three times.

Then commence with the following strokes. From the superior dorsal border of the greater trochanter follow the ilio-tibial band, ending the
stroke over the insertion of the lateral hamstring with a hook-on (Figure
17-25). Facing the head of the patient, surround the greater trochanter

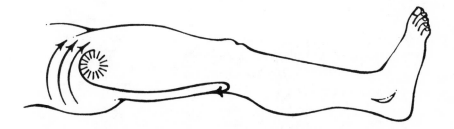

Figure 17-25. Lower extremity.

with small ellipsoid strokes. Beginning distally, follow the ilio-tibial band for its upper two-thirds and finish the stroke around the greater trochanter. Give ellipsoid strokes in the space between the greater trochanter up to the iliac spine. Support the leg with the free hand from the lateral side. Stroke between the semi-membranosis and the semi-tendinosis down the lower third with a stretch hook-on technique at the end of the stroke, near its insertion (Figure 17-26).

Bimanually stroke both hamstrings from the gluteal fold to their distal portion, where the hands are turned outward at the end of the stroke to provide a stretch of the tendons at their insertion. (Never use this stroke if varicosity exists.) Stroke from the distal gastrocnemius where the belly begins to the knee, turning the hands outward at the top of the gastrocnemius. This movement comes through the arms, not the fingers. Stay in the groove, stroking gently. Provide widening of the knee by using both hands to provide a bilateral stretch or widening technique to the popliteal space, stretching first the hamstrings then the gastrocnemius (see Figure 17-27).

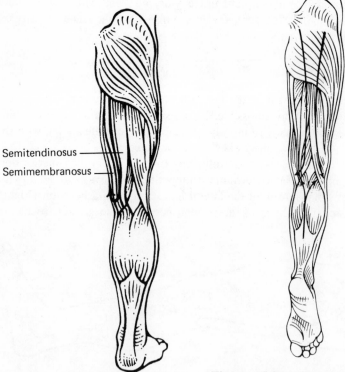

Semitendinosus
Semimembranosus

Figure 17-26. Lower extremity.

Figure 17-27. Lower extremity and foot.

Lower Extremity and Foot

Bimanually stroke the Achilles tendon, working from proximal to distal, beginning just distal to the belly of the muscle, pulling to the back of the heel. The hand should help to flex the foot slightly. Stroke the peroneous longus and brevis, around the malleolus toward the dorsum of the foot. Stabilize the leg with the other hand. Do the same for the posterior tibialis. Bimanually stroke down both sides.

Figure 17-28 illustrates a posterior view of these strokes. Figure 17-29 illustrates the lateral view of the above strokes; and Figure 17-30, the medial view.

If arthritis is present in the knee do not do the following strokes. Face the patient. With one hand, use short strokes which hook under the border of the patella, while stabilizing the patient's leg with the other hand. Begin medially and work to the lateral knee. The fingers should be bent, trying to reach under the patella. First do the superior aspect of the patella; then stroke around the inferior aspect of the patella,

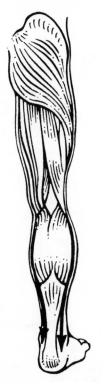

Figure 17-28. Posterior view, lower extremity and foot.

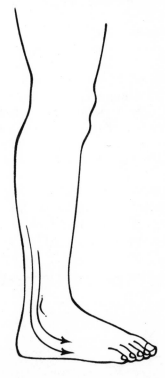

Figure 17-29. Lateral view, lower extremity and foot.

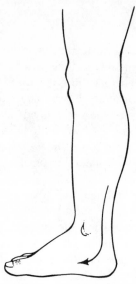

Figure 17-30. Medial view, lower extremity and foot.

stroking toward it using the other hand. Using a pivot-like stroke in which the heel of the hand acts as the pivot to stroke around the patella. First stroke across the top of the patella from medial to lateral. Then below, stroke from the medial to the lateral aspect (Figure 17-31). Stabilizing the foot with one hand, apply little strokes across the front of the ankle joint, dorsi flexing the ankle at the same time. Provide short little strokes between the metatarsophalangeal joints, proximal to distal, medial to lateral. The dorsum of the foot is not treated. Apply deep little strokes just in front of the heel from the arch around the side of the foot, always starting laterally and working medially. Do the same to the medial side of the foot, going the other way around. Then give short strokes across the heel (Figures 17-32, 17-33).

Provide deep stroking of the plantar aspect of the foot with long

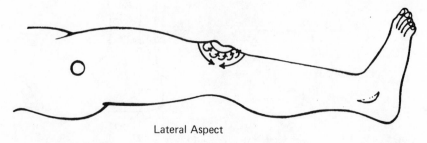

Lateral Aspect

Figure 17-31. Pivot-like strokes to the patella.

Note: Not All Strokes Are Illustrated.

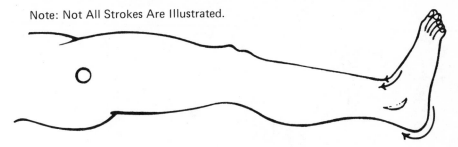

Figure 17-32. Foot, lateral view.

strokes which cover the longitudinal arch from the heel up to the meta-tarsophalangeal joint. Then stroke the lateral and medial borders of the foot. Repeat this on the lateral aspect of the plantar surface. Apply medial plantar stroking across the muscle fibers at a right angle to the longitudinal arch.

Bilaterally stretch both the top and the bottom of the foot with a rolling motion of the hands. Go up and out on the proximal part of the foot. Pronate the hands with pressure and continue the same technique to the distal part of the foot. Then supinate the hands and forearms (Figures 17-34 to 17-36).

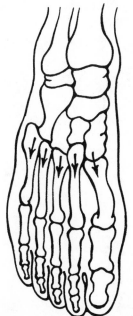

Figure 17-33. Foot, frontal view.

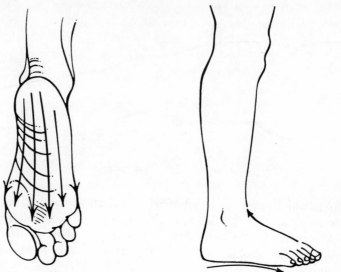

Figure 17-34. Stretching the foot.   **Figure 17-35.** Stretching the foot.

Face

Stand behind the patient so that the patient's head leans against the operator. Using bimanual strokes across the forehead, stroke three times from the hairline until just above the eyebrows, moving towards the

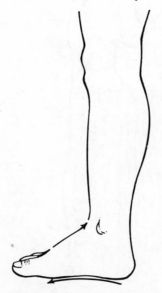

Figure 17-36. Stretching the foot.

temple. Short hook-on strokes from the midline to the temple, starting on the involved side are given. Do all of one side of the face and then the other.

Give very soft pulls into the hairline of the temple from the lateral side of the eye. Have your hand well anchored. Follow the upper eyebrow, stroking medial to lateral to the temple. Repeat the same, following the lower rim of the eyebrow. Give similar strokes just below the eye. Give short strokes upward between the eyes. Pull from the involved side to the other side over the bridge of the nose. Give "bimanual" widening of the nose by stroking from the center to each side. Bimanually stroke over the zygotmaticus working from just under the eyes toward the mandible, stroking from the front to the back with four strokes (see Figures 17-37, 17-38). Finish with the balancing stroke down the back.

Table 17-1 and Figures 17-39 to 17-53 compare acupuncture points and overlapping anatomical sites used in the Bindegewebsmassage system that claim relief of symptoms for the same disabilities. A careful study in which areas treated with Bindegewebsmassage are compared with acupuncture as done by the Japanese and Chinese seems to confirm the relationship between the two systems.

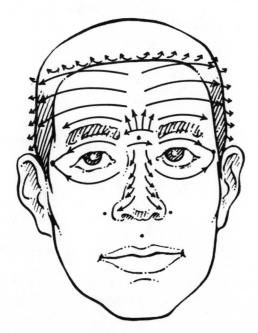

Figure 17-37. Face. frontal view.

Table 17-1

A Comparison of Bindegewebsmassage and Acupuncture Points

ACUPUNCTURE POINT	ANATOMICAL SITE	DISABILITIES
B-40	At the center of the popliteal fossa	Knee pain
B-60	Midpoint between the posterior margin of the lateral malleolus and the Achilles tendon	Diseases of the ankle joint and surrounding soft tissue
GB-20	Midpoint of a line joining the tip of the mastoid process to the posterior midline in the groove between the trapezius and the sternocleidomastoid	Headache Hypertension
GB-21	Midway between C$_7$ and acromion process	Shoulder and back pain Upper extremity impairment
GB-30	One-third of the distance from the greater trochanter to the base of the coccyx	Lower extremity circulatory disorders
GB-34	Anterior to the neck of the fibula	Lower extremity disorders Knee pain
LI-11	Radial end of fold of fully flexed elbow	Disorders of the elbow joint and surrounding soft tissue

Table 17-1 Continued

ACUPUNCTURE POINT	ANATOMICAL SITE	DISABILITIES
LI-15	In the depression of the acromion in the center of the deltoid muscle when the arm is abducted to 90°	Pain and impaired movement of elbow and arm. Disorders of the shoulder and surrounding soft tissue
Special Point 1 Yin-tang	At the glabella, midway between the medial margins of the eyebrows	Disorders of the nose Headache
Special Point 2 Tai-yang	At the temple, one cun directly posterior to the midpoint of a line joining the lateral canthus of the eye and the lateral margin of the eyebrow	Facial paralysis

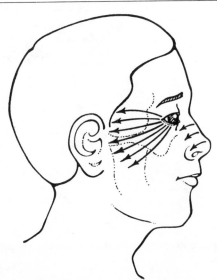

Figure 17-38. Face, lateral view.

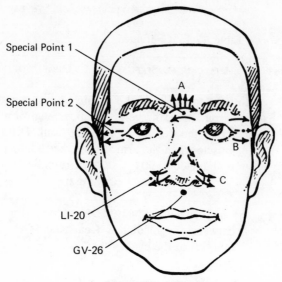

Special Point 1

Special Point 2

LI-20

GV-26

A—Corner of Eye over Nose
B—Temple Strokes to Hairline
C—Stretching the Nose

Figure 17-39. Comparison of acupuncture points and anatomical sites used in Bindegewebsmassage. Frontal view of face.

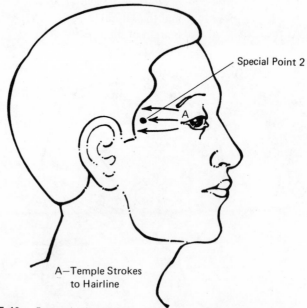

Special Point 2

A—Temple Strokes
to Hairline

Figure 17-40. Lateral view of face showing temple strokes to hairline.

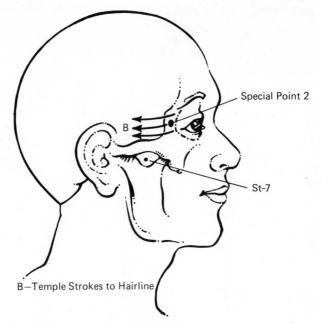

Figure 17-41. Lateral view of face.

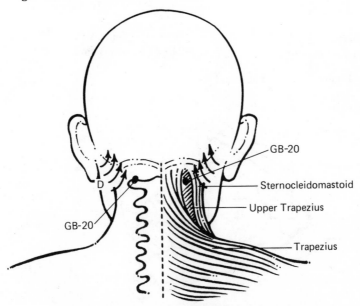

D—Stroke on Posterior Skull along Ligamentum Nuchae to Mastoid Process

Figure 17-42. Back and neck.

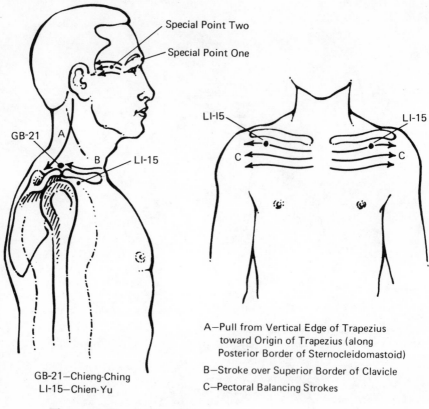

A—Pull from Vertical Edge of Trapezius
    toward Origin of Trapezius (along
    Posterior Border of Sternocleidomastoid)

B—Stroke over Superior Border of Clavicle

C—Pectoral Balancing Strokes

GB-21—Chieng-Ching
LI-15—Chien-Yu

Figure 17-43. Back and neck.

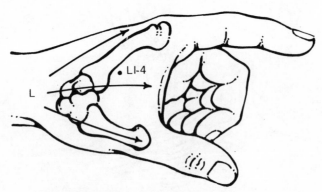

L—Hand Strokes between Metacarpals
LI-4—Ho-Ku
P-6—Nei-Kuan
SI-3—Hou-Chi

Figure 17-44. Hand.

172

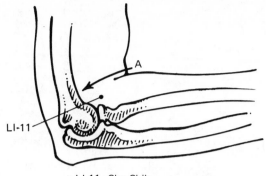

LI-11—Chu-Chih
A—Stretching of the Elbow

Figure 17-45. Elbow.

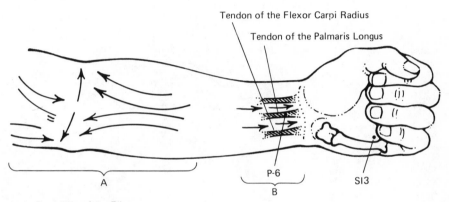

Tendon of the Flexor Carpi Radius

Tendon of the Palmaris Longus

P-6

A

B

SI3

A—Stretching of the Elbow
B—Strokes over the Flexor Carpi Radius,
  Palmaris Longus, and Flexor Carpi Ulnaris

Figure 17-46. Forearm.

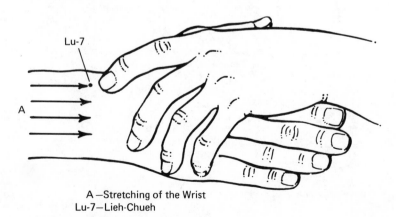

Lu-7

A

A—Stretching of the Wrist
Lu-7—Lieh-Chueh

Figure 17-47. Wrist.

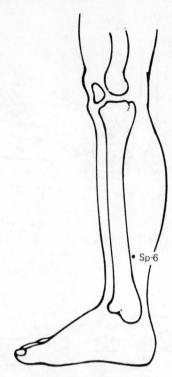

Figure 17-48. Leg. Sp-6—San-yin-chiao

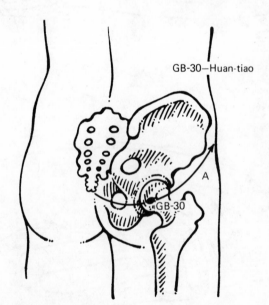

GB-30—Huan-tiao

A—Pelvic stroke from anal fold along ischial tuberosity

Figure 17-49. Pelvic stroke.

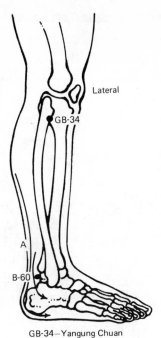

GB-34—Yangung Chuan
B-60—Kunlun
A—Stretching the heel

Figure 17-50. Heel.

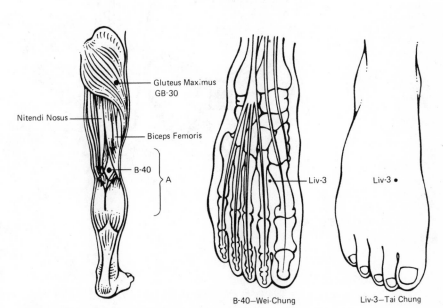

B-40—Wei-Chung

Liv-3—Tai Chung

A —Strokes from dorsal seat fold to popliteal fossa
and strokes along gastrocnemius into popliteal fossa

Figure 17-51. Leg and foot.

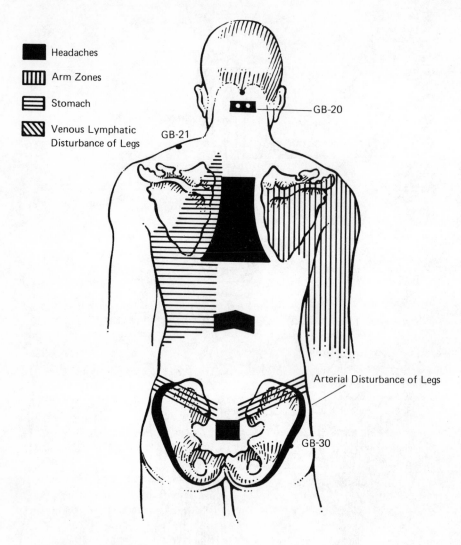

Figure 17-52.

Chapter 18

Reflexology

Although acupuncture is seldom given on the bottom of the foot, the Chinese feel that the total body is reflected in the ear, eye, palm of the hand, and bottom of the foot.

Recently, a great deal of emphasis has been placed on treating disorders of the entire body by treating the bottom of the foot with rather deep pressure in certain key spots.

Centuries before Head identified viscero-cutaneous and cutaneo-visceral reflex effects in the 1800's, the Chinese had identified sensitive areas on the bottom of the feet. Using finger pressure because needles were too painful, they treated specific areas on the feet to normalize physiological functions in the human body.

Dr. William H. Fitzgerald rediscovered this Chinese method of foot massage and brought it to the attention of the medical world in the United States in 1913, calling it "Zone Therapy." It continues to be taught by descendants of Eunice D. Ingham (Mrs. Fred Stopfel), a major advocate of this technique.[1]

The technique for administration of this form of massage consists of compression, using the thumbs to apply firm pressure. By doing compression over the entire foot, tender areas will indicate where concen-

[1] The purpose of this discussion is to bring Zone Therapy to the attention of the reader. For greater detail, consult Eunice D. Ingham, *Stories the Feet Can Tell* (Rochester: Eunice D. Ingham, 1959).

The illustrations used here are not those from Ingham's text, but come from *The Massage Book* by George Downing, illustrated by Anne Kent Rush (N.Y.: Random House, and Berkeley, Calif.: The Bookworks, 1974), pp. 151-52.

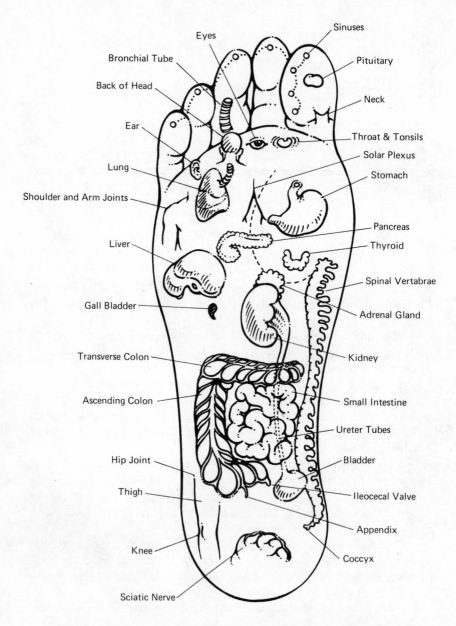

Figure 18-1. Right foot, bottom view.

178

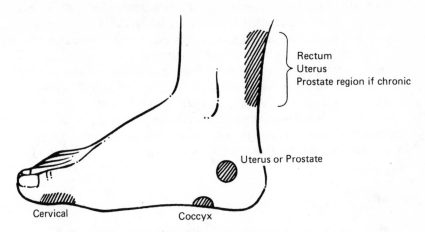

Figure 18-2. Right foot, lateral view.

tration of treatment should be given. Twenty minutes is an adequate amount of time to treat both feet. Care should be taken to stay within the person's pain tolerance level. The one being treated should be told that pressure needs to be firm but not overly painful.

Skilled and experienced thumbs can palpate areas of tightness or swelling on the foot. All references concerning Zone Therapy agree as to which areas relate to various parts of the body. Attempts to explain

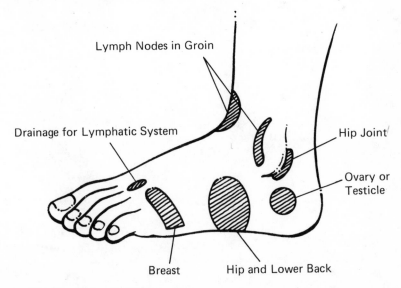

Figure 18-3. Left foot.

physiologically why Zone Therapy is effective are as difficult as explaining any of the other methods referred to in this text. The term "energy flow" in the human body is often used in recent research findings to describe such phenomena. (See Chapter 6.)

Other massage systems maintain that the connective tissue and the lymph system throughout the body are the vehicles for energy circuits of a nature not yet analyzed by either Eastern or Western medical science. It is the author's belief that when the explanation is found for the effects of acupuncture, the foundations for the physiological effects of Zone Therapy and Bindegewebsmassage (connective tissue massage) will also be discovered.

Summary

Although this discussion is brief, the explanation plus the illustrations give the reader an idea of the procedures. It is recommended, however, that further course work on this topic be undertaken if the operator intends to become skillful in the use of reflexology.

Chapter 19

James Cyriax

James Cyriax thinks that the most potent form of massage is deep friction: [1]

> The principle governing the treatment of muscles during the acute or chronic stage is the same. The endeavor must be to prevent the continued adherence of unwanted young fibrous tissue in recent cases, or to rupture adherent scar tissue in long-standing cases. To stretch out a muscle does not widen the distance between its fibres; on the contrary, during stretching they lie more closely. Whereas, then, for the rupture of adherent scars about a joint, forced movement is required; interfibrillary adhesions in muscle can be broken, not by stretching, but by forcibly broadening the muscle out. Particularly is this true of the fibres of attachment of muscle into bone, where the vicinity of stationary tissue restricts the mobility of adjacent muscle. *Thus, deep transverse frictions restore mobility to muscle in the same way a manipulation frees a joint. Indeed, the action of deep transverse friction may be summed up as affording a mobilization that passive stretching or active exercises cannot achieve.*
>
> After the friction has restored a full range of painless broadening to the muscle belly, this added mobility must be maintained. To this end, the patient should perform a series of active contractions with the joint placed in a position that fully relaxes the affected muscle, i.e., the position that allows the greatest

[1] Cyriax, James and Russell, Gillean, *Textbook of Orthopaedic Medicine*, Volume II, 9th ed. (London: Baillière Tindall, 1977. Distributed by Macmillan Inc., New York.)

broadening. Strong resisted movements should be avoided until the scar has consolidated itself; otherwise, started too soon, they tend to strain the healing breach again. Athletes in particular must not return to full sport too early.

TYPES OF MANUAL TREATMENT

Deep Effleurage

This technique serves to relieve congestion. Swelling is treated in many situations by upward stroking of sufficient depth to remove it. The chief indications for effleurage are oedema and traumatic periostitis.

Oedema

Whether the oedema appears as the result of an injury, of the removal of a plaster cast from the lower limb or of venous thrombosis or is of the type known as angioneurotic, effleurage is usually indicated for its diminution or removal. A crepe bandage should be applied tightly at the end of each session and kept on until the next session. The massage should be given daily, sometimes more often. In the treatment of oedema due to heart failure, phlebitis, nephritis or lymphatic obstruction caused by carcinomatous invasion, massage is only a temporary palliative. The oedema about an infected area must not be treated by massage, and hereditary oedema of the leg (Milroy's disease) and oedema due to filaria (elephantiasis) are not benefited. The oedema that always occurs after an amputation, especially at the lower limb, should be treated not by massage but by continuous pressure bandaging, tightening several times a day.[2]

Traumatic Periostitis

Since the periosteum is attached to a motionless structure—bone—the formation of adherent scars is harmless. Deep friction is, therefore, never required. The periosteum is painful because it is swollen, and no more need be done than to reduce the swelling by firm, but not painful, deep effleurage, given daily. If a subperiosteal haematoma is present, aspiration will much hasten the patient's recovery, since blood is absorbed very slowly thence.[3]

[2] *Ibid.*, p. 9.
[3] *Ibid.*

Deep Friction

The most potent form of massage is deep friction. By this means alone, massage can reach structures far below the surface of the body. Since the source of pain in patients for whom manual methods are required so often lie in muscle, tendon or ligament, whether as the result of injury or repeated strain, a penetrating technique is clearly essential if such tissues are to be affected. . . .

When mobility is to be maintained at, or restored to, those moving parts which from their nature or position are apt to develop adhesions or scarring, deep friction is often the method of choice, either alone (as in the case of tendons) or in association with passive movements (for some ligamentous lesions) or with active movement without tension or the healing breach (for minor muscular ruptures). An important part of the [operator's] knowledge consists in choosing and applying whichever type of therapeutic movement is best adapted to the patient's disorder.[4]

Mode of Action of Deep Massage

A penetrating technique is required in the treatment by massage of deep-seated lesions. Given properly, deep friction has a dual effect. It induces (1) traumatic hyperaemia and (2) movement.

1. *Traumatic Hyperaemia* Enhancement of the blood supply diminishes pain. Apparently it acts by increasing the speed of destruction of Lewis's P-substance, the factor responsible for pain. Heat and counterirritants soothe for the duration of their application, also as the result of similar enhancement of blood-flow. They have no lasting effect upon the type of lesion under discussion, because no other change than the circulatory is secured. Deep massage results in a more lasting hyperaemia and it appears to be in this way that the friction, though in itself painful, is found at the end of the session to have allayed the symptoms for a while. In other words, deep massage given to the lesion itself affords temporary analgesia, and during this period treatment can be given that pain would otherwise have prevented.

2. *Movement* By moving the painful structure to and fro, it is freed from adhesions both actually present and in the process of formation. Clearly massage applied parallel to the length of a structure follows the course of the blood and lymph vessels,

4 *Ibid.,* pp. 9-10.

whereas transverse friction does not. Hence longitudinal frictions merely move blood and lymph along, whereas *transverse friction moves the tissue itself.* In most conditions, there is nothing wrong with the circulation, hence there is no advantage in trying to alter it. I regard the lasting benefit that so often follows massage in muscular, tendinous and ligamentous lesions as accruing from the application of therapeutic movement to the affected part.[5]

Deep Massage for Muscular Lesions

The main function of muscle is to contract. As it does it broadens. Hence full mobility in broadening out must be maintained or restored in muscles that have been the seat of inflammation, whether caused by one or by repeated strains. Resolution by fibrosis is occurring or has already occurred. The effect of deep transverse friction clearly consists in mobilizing the muscle, i.e., separating the adhesions between individual muscle fibres that are restricting movement. If passive restoration of full mobility of a muscle is followed by adequate active use, these adhesions do not re-form; cure results.[6]

Deep Massage for Ligamentous Lesions

In recent cases, after any oedema that may be present has been removed by effleurage, the site of the minor tear in the ligament should receive some minutes' friction. The purpose is to disperse blood clot or effusion here, to move the ligament to and fro over subjacent bone in imitation of its normal behavior (thus maintaining its mobility) and to numb it enough to facilitate movement afterwards. The least strength of friction which achieves these results is called for. Hence, when friction is started during the first day or two after a sprain, the ligament need be moved only a few times. One minute's treatment thus suffices, since as yet there are no unwanted adhesions to break down. But it may well take ten to twenty minutes' effleurage and gentle friction to enable the patient to accept the one minute's valid treatment—actually moving the damaged tissue. When the lesion becomes less severe and tenderness is abating, friction maintained with increasing strength for five, ten, then fifteen minutes is called for.

When acute traumatic arthritis is present at a joint such as the knee, muscle spasm so limits movement at the joint that it is impossible to maintain the mobility of a ligament in the usual way,

[5] *Ibid.,* pp. 10-11.

[6] *Ibid.,* p. 11.

i.e., by moving the bones to and fro under it. In such a case the only . . . alternative is to use the human finger to move the ligament to and fro over the bone in imitation of its normal behavior. This is the very mobilization that transverse friction achieves, provided that it is given deeply enough to reach the injured fibres of the ligament.

In chronic cases deep friction is given to fibrous structures such as ligaments in preparation for manipulation. The friction thins out the scar tissue by which the fibrous structure is held abnormally adherent, and so numbs it that rupture by forcing becomes tolerable. However, in the case of the dorsal ligaments at the wrist, the coronary ligaments at the knee and the femoral extent of the medial collateral ligament at the knee and the sacrococcygeal ligament, the massage is itself the mobilizing agent and no forcing of movement follows.[7]

Deep Massage for Tendinous Lesions

In acute and chronic teno-synovitis the way deep massage acts is somewhat different. On logical grounds it has been widely held that teno-synovitis, being as a result of overuse, should not be treated by further friction. Nevertheless this is the very condition in which massage achieves some of its quickest and most brilliant results. The phenomenon of crepitus proves that roughening of the gliding surfaces occurs. The fact that slitting up the sheath of the tendon at open operation is immediately curative shows that it was the movement between the close-fitting sheath and the tendon that set up the pain. Hence it would appear that manual rolling of the tendon sheath to and fro against the tendon serves to smooth the gliding surfaces off again. While the causative overuse was longitudinal friction, the curative is transverse.

In those tendons that lack a sheath, deep massage acts by breaking up scar tissue at the insertion of the tendon into bone or within its substance. Since no sheath exists, there is no reason to suppose that some slight roughening of the surface of the tendon would cause symptoms. Deep friction provides the only method whereby the [operator] can bring lasting relief in these cases. The alternative is local infiltration with hydrocortisone, which disinflames the scar, but leaves this still in existence. Hydrocortisone, when it succeeds, is a quicker method of securing relief, but it is followed by a higher frequency of recurrence on account of the persistence of the scar.

Since the cause of teno-synovitis and tendinitis is overuse, no exercises follow. Splintage is quite unnecessary; the patient merely told to avoid any exertion that hurts.[8]

[7] *Ibid.*, p. 12.

[8] *Ibid.*, p. 13.

MASSAGE WITH CREAMS

When deep friction is given, the [operator's] finger and the patient's skin must move as one. The application of any cream, ointment or powder, or even previous heat leading to local sweating, makes the skin slippery and must be avoided. But for centuries laymen's expectations have been periodically aroused that rubbing in this or that cream or liniment has a curative value. The effect postulated is local, not systemic as in mercurial inunction for syphilis. Naturally, it makes not the slightest difference to the deeper tissues what is or is not rubbed into the skin; for all agents that penetrate are absorbed by the blood in the cutaneous capillary system and removed. Counter-irritation results, of course, and the patient may feel a pleasant glow, but it is probable that, by drawing more of the available blood towards the skin, the flow through the underlying tissues becomes diminished for the time being. But minor ephemeral ischaemia is not likely to do good, since analgesic measures rely on an increase in the local circulation.

The usefulness of rubbing in any cream, liniment or embrocation, however convincingly advertised to the layman and, even more assiduously, to health professionals, is worth stressing. Thousands of pounds are wasted on these remedies by laymen and National Health Service alike. Such striking claims were made twenty years ago by Moss for a massage cream containing adrenaline that the Empire Rheumatism Council set up a subcommittee to investigate. It reported that whether adrenaline was present in the cream or not made no real difference to the result, and that none of the systemic effects of adrenaline was noted.[9]

Those interested in Cyriax's techniques should consult his complete book, *Textbook of Orthopaedic Medicine.*

[9] *Ibid.,* p. 14.

Chapter 20

Albert J. Hoffa

This discussion does not include a *complete* translation of Hoffa's text, for much of it would not be applicable today. However, a complete translation has been made, and the techniques described here closely follow the literal translation.[1]

Hoffa uses what he describes as the anatomical method for the different parts of the body, following the larger vessels, and selecting specific muscles or muscle groups to be massaged in order.

He states that the following general considerations should be kept in mind. The force should not be rude or brutal; all manipulations should be gentle and "light-handed" so that the patient feels as little pain as possible. No point should be treated for too long. Hoffa's text does not advocate any massage for over 15 minutes, even for a total body massage.[2]

No massage should be done through clothing. The part to be massaged should be as relaxed as possible. The joints should be kept in mid-position so that tension of capsule ligaments and tendons is at a minimum.

---

[1] With the help of Miss Ruth Friedlander, the author translated Hoffa's book into English. Passages quoted in this chapter are from that translation, but the page numbers refer to Hoffa's text in case the reader should wish to refer to the original.

[2] Max Bohm's book (*Massage: Its Principles and Technic*, translated by Elizabeth Gould. W. B. Saunders Co., Philadelphia, 1913) which is representative of Hoffa's technique as interpreted by Bohm, states, however, that up to three-quarters of an hour can be taken for massage of the whole body.

If the hands are rough, a lubricant should be used. Hoffa maintains that if the part to be massaged is covered with hair it should be shaved. The operator should start with the healthy part and massage gradually toward the injured area, always stroking with the venous flow.

Effleurage should be used for beginning and ending the massage as well as between all other strokes. If the part is covered by thick heavy fascia, effleurage is not deep enough and greater pressure is needed. Therefore, the knuckles must be used. Pressure is not continuous, but swells up and down, starting lightly and becoming stronger, then decreasing again. The hand should not stick to the part but glide over it lightly. If the hands are moist, they should be washed with alcohol and rubbed with salicylic powder.

HOFFA'S EFFLEURAGE TECHNIQUES

Light and Deep Stroking

The following description of effleurage is applied to both light and deep stroking; the deep stroking differs only in the amount of pressure applied:

> The hand is applied as closely as possible to the part. It glides on it, distally to proximally. . . . With the broad part of the hand use the ball of the thumb and little fingers to stroke out the muscle masses, and at the same time, slide along at the edge of the muscle with finger tips to take care of all larger vessels; stroke upward.[3]

Knuckling

Knuckling is a stroke particularly associated with the Hoffa techniques. In describing it he says:

> If the part to be treated is covered by thick fascia, effleurage (as described above) is not deep enough. You need greater pressure, therefore the convex dorsal sides of the first interphalangeal joints must be used. Clench the fist in strong plantar flexion, knuckles in the peripheral end stroking upwards, gradually bringing the hand from plantar to dorsal flexion. Pressure is not continuous, swelling up and down, starting lightly and becoming stronger, then decreasing again. The hand must not adhere to the

---

[3] Hoffa, p. 2.

part, but should glide over it lightly. Knuckling should only be used where there is enough room for the hand to be applied.[4]

Circular Effleurage

Hoffa often refers to what he calls "circular effleurage." In regard to circular effleurage of the fingers he writes:

> To do circular effleurage of each single finger, stroke around each finger from its point to its base, with strokes that cover each other like the shingles of a roof. Execute these strokes with the tip of the index and middle finger of the right hand, held in opposition to each other, while you lay the volar surface on your own left hand underneath the fingers on which you are working to support them. To make this stroke more vigorous use the tips of your two thumbs.[5]

To adapt circular effleurage to the arm, he says, "Begin on the forearm, stroking around the joint and doing strokes in such a manner that they always end up in either the biceps or triceps group. While one hand supports, the other hand massages." [6]

Thumb Stroking

Hoffa uses an alternate thumb stroking on the foot. He describes its use on the dorsum of the foot by saying, "Massage each tendon sheath by means of strokes of the thumb, alternating from the base of the toes up over the ankle joint." [7]

Alternate-Hand Stroking

No description of alternate effleurage stroking could be found other than the use of alternate *thumb* stroking on the foot.

Others

Hoffa mentions the use of simultaneous stroking and the use of one-hand stroking, but does not describe the use of the one hand over the other for deeper pressure.[8]

[4] Hoffa, p. 2.
[5] Hoffa, p. 51.
[6] Hoffa, p. 58.
[7] Hoffa, p. 62.
[8] Hoffa, pp. 29, 32.

HOFFA'S PETRISSAGE TECHNIQUES

One-Hand Petrissage

Place the hand around the part so that the muscle-masses are caught between the fingers and thumb as in a pair of tongs. By lifting the muscle-mass from the bone, "squeeze it out," progressing centripetally. On flat surfaces where this petrissage is not possible, Hoffa does a stroke using a flat hand instead of picking up the muscle. This type of kneading is recommended for use on small limbs.[9]

Two-Hand Petrissage

Apply both hands obliquely to the direction of the muscle fibers. The thumbs are opposed to the rest of the fingers. This manipulation starts peripherally and proceeds centripetally, following the direction of the muscle fibers. The hand that goes first tries to pick the muscle from the bone, moving back and forth in a zigzag path. The hand that follows proceeds likewise, "gripping back and forth." This progressive movement is made easier by doing most of the work from the shoulder.[10] On flat surfaces where this petrissage is not possible Hoffa does the stroke using a *flat* hand, instead of picking up the muscle.

Two-Finger Petrissage

Over parts where muscle bellies are flat rather than round, and one cannot grasp hold with a full hand (such as the back, or over places where muscles are overlaid by strong fascias) the most useful kind of petrissage is the two-finger petrissage. Grasp the part between thumb and forefinger. Press it out by making little circular movements from the shoulder, making the fingers move the skin along with the rest of the movement. Some people refer to this as "creepy crawl" or "creepy mouse," but neither term connotes relaxation. This author prefers Hoffa's terminology, "two-finger petrissage."

Friction

In describing friction Hoffa says:

> Put the thumb in the neighborhood of the part to be massaged, setting the index finger of the right hand on the skin

[9] Hoffa, p. 9.
[10] Hoffa, pp. 9-10.

of the part, more or less vertically. Penetrate into the depth, not by moving the points of the fingers on the skin, but by moving the skin under the fingers.

In going deep, describe small flat ellipsoids with the point of the index finger. These follow each other as quickly and consecutively as possible. The finger joints and wrist are to be kept almost stiff and the elbow joint only makes small excursions. The main movement is made from the shoulder joint.[11]

He uses the index finger of the left hand to intersperse effleurage with the friction strokes.

In reference to the use of other fingers or part of the hand for friction, Hoffa refers only to the thumb, using it either to fit better to some anatomical part or to rest the forefinger. He also suggests using both thumb and index finger to do friction at the same time.

Hoffa uses the *thumb*, the *index finger, or both* for friction.

Tapotement

In describing tapotement, Hoffa says:

Both hands are held vertically above the part to be treated in a position that is midway between pronation and supination. Bringing them into supination, the abducted fingers are hit against the body with not too much force and with great speed and elasticity. Fingers and wrists remain as stiff as possible but the shoulder joint comes into play all the more actively." [12]

Hoffa used this hacking stroke routinely with all back massages.

Vibration

Hoffa says that vibration may be done either with the points of the fingers or with the hand lying flat. The forearm is at right angles to the upper arm. The whole forearm is brought into a rhythmical trembling movement from the elbow joint, but the wrist and finger joints are kept as stiff as possible. Even though he describes the technique, he feels that it is better to use a mechanical vibrator.[13]

Massage of the Upper Extremity

In describing stroking and petrissage of the limbs, Hoffa begins with the right forearm, dividing it into two groups, the flexors and the

[11] Hoffa, pp. 11-12.

[12] Hoffa, p. 14.

[13] Hoffa, pp. 15-17.

extensors. The patient sits facing the operator, with the arm in a neutral position between flexion and abduction, and the elbow at an obtuse angle with the radial side upward. The patient should be as relaxed as possible. Three or four times is enough of each stroke to accomplish the purpose of effleurage.

After stroking out the muscles, petrissage is given. As in effleurage the muscle groups should be kept strictly in mind. First the extensors are kneaded, starting at the wrist and ending at the elbow. The hand lifts up the extensors between the thumb and the other four fingers, kneading them centripetally. Once having arrived at the elbow joint, intersperse a few effleurage strokes about three times before undertaking a kneading of the flexors in a similar manner.

The upper arm is divided into three muscle groups. Group one includes the biceps, brachialis and coracobrachialis. The second group is the triceps muscle alone; the third division is the deltoid, which is divided into two parts, the back and the front. Massage of the upper arm begins with the stroking and kneading of the biceps group. The triceps are then considered. One applies the hand to the back of the arm, beginning just below the olecranon, gliding upward in the external bicipital sulcus and then on to the outer edge of the deltoid and into the auxiliary pit. The posterior part of the deltoid is massaged before the anterior portion and the massage to the upper extremity is finished.

In massage of the hand, Hoffa does a circular effleurage of each of the fingers. In doing this he strokes around each finger from its point to its base with strokes that cover each other like the shingles of a roof. He executes these strokes with the tip of the index and middle fingers of the right hand, held in opposition to each other, while he lays the volar surface of his own left hand underneath the fingers on which he is working to support them. These strokes he refers to as "shingle strokes. " [14]

For petrissage of the fingers, he takes hold of the soft part from both sides between the thumb and forefinger of his two hands and picks them up off the bone (as best he can), while moving along the skin and describing small circles, squeezing and progressing from the point of one finger to the base of the other in a zigzag fashion. The rest of the hand is done with alternate thumb stroking from the metacarpophalangeal joint to the wrist, and knuckling is done to the palmar fascia. The message of the foot is very similar.[15]

[14] Hoffa, pp. 23-62.
[15] Hoffa, pp. 51-62.

Massage of the Lower Extremity

Hoffa mentions turning the patient when treating both front and back of the lower extremity. (This technique is no longer widely practiced and it is felt that the patient should not be disturbed any more than is absolutely necessary.) Place the patient either on his back or prone and adapt all techniques so that anterior and posterior aspects of the lower extremity are treated from one position.

Hoffa shows an illustration of the patient seated, with his leg in the operator's lap.[16] This author doubts that Hoffa, were he alive today, would recommend a position where support of the limb is so poor.

For massage of the lower extremity, the patient is seated, with his leg in the operator's lap.[17] The hip is in inward rotation, the knee slightly bent for massage of the outer muscles, and the leg is rotated outward to reach the medial muscle groups.

Beginning with the lower leg, he divides it into four groups: first, the tibialis anticus with the extensors digitorum, communis longus, and hallucis longus; second, the peroneal muscles; third, the outer half of the calf muscles; fourth, the inner half of the calf muscles with the tibialis posticus, flexor hallucis longus and flexor digitorum communis longus. Taking the above named groups in order, they are effleuraged and petrissaged. On the first group the usual effleurage is followed by a few strokes done with the knuckles, due to the strong crural fascia. Two-finger petrissage is also used on this group. At the knee joint, intersperse a few effleurage strokes and begin to knead again. The peroneal group is covered in like manner. The last two groups are massaged with the usual effleurage and one-hand petrissage.

Massage of the thigh is divided into the quadriceps; adductors; tensor fascia lata; biceps; semitendinosus and semimembranosus; and, the glutei. For massage of the quadriceps and adductor group the patient lies on his back, and for the tensor fascia lata he lies on his side. For the remaining parts he lies on his stomach. All groups are given effleurage and petrissage in the prescribed manner, with knuckling over the tensor fascia lata. The glutei are divided into two groups, considering the oblique direction of the fibers that run from the trochanter towards the iliac crest and those from the greater trochanter toward the sacrum and then toward the iliac crest. The operator is seated on the side of the patient opposite the part being massaged. Both sections are given effleurage and petrissage.

[16] Hoffa, p. 23.
[17] Hoffa, p. 23.

Massage of the Back

The back massage first considers the long, back muscles, with the stroke beginning at the limit between the back and neck. The stroke progresses downward, leaving the spinous processes free, with the tips of the first and second fingers performing most of the stroke (Figure 20-1). As the hands reach the sacrum, they diverge laterally from each other and follow the course of the iliac crest to the inguinal region. There the stroke is ended and the upward stroke begins. The stroke returns in a similar fashion to the sacrum and proceeds upward to the hairline (Figure 20-2) where the hands glide along the neck laterally to arrive at the sternoclavicular joint. After several repetitions of these strokes knuckle effleurage follows to affect the deeper tissues. Two-finger petrissage is then given to the long muscles of the back. The fingerpaint patterns illustrate direction of the strokes and the area covered.

The latissimus dorsi is then effleuraged from origin to insertion (Figure 20-3). The trapezius is divided into three groups in accordance with the three-fold fiber direction (Figure 20-4). Each group is considered separately and given effleurage. This is contrary to the common opinion that Hoffa stroked the trapezius with an alternate effleurage

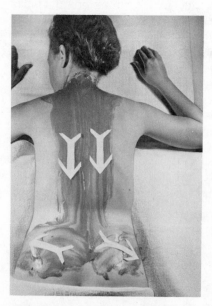
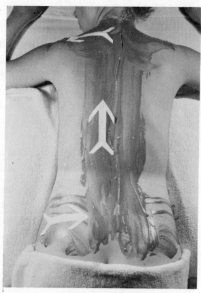

Figure 20-1. Erector spinae group. **Figure 20-2.** Erector spinae group.

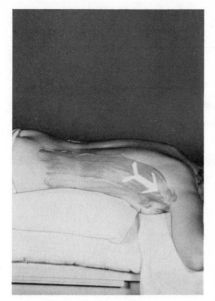

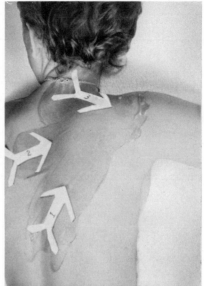

Figure 20-3.   Latissimus dorsi.   **Figure 20-4.**   Trapezius.

stroke, but the description given here is upheld by Bohm.[18] Petrissage, using the flat hand, is given on the latissimus dorsi and lower and middle trapezius. Tapotement in the form of hacking is given after muscle groups have been effleuraged and petrissaged. All of one side of the back is done before moving to the opposite side of the table to massage the other side of the back.

SUMMARY

The fact that Hoffa was one of the earliest to describe massage in a text, coupled with the accuracy of his descriptions, may account for the fact that his five fundamental strokes are still done today much as they were then, although the pattern or area of the stroke may vary greatly. Principles of positioning have changed since the days when Hoffa put the patient's foot comfortably in his lap to work on it. There is no denying that Hoffa's methods are still used throughout America today, although those who use them are often unaware that they were written in German by Hoffa. It is hoped this text will enlighten many and give Hoffa the credit that is most certainly due him.

18 Bohm, p. 73.

Chapter 21

Mary McMillan

Mary McMillan considers massage as the manipulation of soft tissues or as movements done upon the body. She divides massage into five fundamental procedures: effleurage, petrissage, friction, tapotement, and vibration.

She believes that the student beginning to use the hands in various forms of manipulation has little difficulty in getting accustomed to dry rubbing. McMillan prefers it, except in cases of excessive scar tissue, of emaciated patients, or after the long use of splints. According to McMillan, cod liver oil or olive oil can be of nutritive value when absorbed through the pores of the skin, and would therefore be good lubricants to use if this type of nutrition is desired. Cocoa butter and lanolin are among the best lubricants, but should be used sparingly. The latter is preferred by some because it is an animal fat.

McMillan's massage was developed from her experience in teaching. Although it is not based on a particular method, she makes reference to J. M. M. Lucas-Championnière, Sir William Bennett, Dr. Weir Mitchell, and Dr. Douglas Graham.[1]

McMillan maintains that one should first define the specific area to be massaged. For instance, in giving massage to the upper extremity begin from the fingertips to just beyond the wrist joint; second, from below the wrist joint to just beyond the elbow joint; and, third, from below the elbow joint to just beyond the shoulder joint.

[1] See Mary McMillan, p. 9.

196

It will be noticed in each subdivision that the stroke is carried from just below the distal joint to just beyond the proximal, the object being to carry the lymph to the proximal glands in order that it may be taken on through the lymphatics, back to the right side of the heart.

An operator who cannot use one hand as well as the other is not only limited in performing the normal operations of the work, but is a 50 per cent worker. Therefore, from the start, one should practice more with the lesser developed hand as soon as some ability to perform certain manipulations is acquired. Great care should be taken to put pressure on the upward stroke, allowing the hand to return to its original position without pressure, but without losing contact with the part being massaged. The fingers of the operator in performing effleurage should be held close together, but not stiffly. Relaxation on the part of the patient is necessary. The greater the facility of the operator to mold the hand into the part being massaged, the better the work will be. This molding is making use to the utmost advantage of the span between the thumb and the fingers *en masse*. Most of the molding process is directed by the thumb and the thenar eminence. No jarring or jerking either at the start or finish of the stroke should ever be felt by the patient.[2]

Concerning treatment time and draping, McMillan says:

There is no hard-and-fast rule, but the following table, stating the approximate length of time for the limbs and trunk, is given as an aid to beginners:

Upper limbs	10 minutes
Lower limbs	15 minutes
Back	7 minutes
Chest	5 minutes
Abdomen	5 minutes

. . . There is no need of exposing any part of the body other than that under treatment at the time. If there is any danger of the patient's taking cold, massage may be given under . . . a light-weight covering. If the patient wears a night-gown, each arm should be taken from the sleeve and replaced when treated. A light-weight but warm shawl is useful to cover the upper part of the back while the lower part is being massaged.[3]

[2] Mary McMillan, *Massage and Therapeutic Exercise*, 3rd ed. (Philadelphia: W. B. Saunders Co.), pp. 20-21.

[3] *Ibid.*, pp. 66-67.

Joint Surfaces

Around joint surfaces pressure is brought to bear upon the underlying structures. In friction of the phalangeal joints the joints of the first and third fingers are manipulated between the finger and thumb of the operator. In the same way the second and fourth fingers receive friction. If friction is given simultaneously to alternate fingers, one hand of the operator is not in the way of the other. Friction is given around the wrist-joint with two or three fingers and thumb. In the lower extremity the toes and ankle-joint receive similar treatment. In cases in which there is excessive scar tissue friction is the most useful form of manipulation to loosen it. . . .

Running frictions are sometimes used to advantage in a case of recovering sciatica. Over the denser area the thenar eminence is used for the circular frictions, starting over the great sciatic notch where the sciatic nerve emerges from the pelvis. These friction movements are carried down the whole area of the terminal endings of the sciatic nerve.[4]

MC MILLAN'S EFFLEURAGE TECHNIQUES

Light and Deep Effleurage

In effleurage, McMillan uses the whole of the palmar surface of the hand. Although light, the stroke is firm and even. The pressure is upward. The fingers are together and the hand is molded to the part. Most of this molding process is directed by the thumb and thenar eminence.[5]

Alternate-Hand Stroking

Concerning alternate-hand stroking, McMillan says, "The third division of the lower extremity is the thigh. Here, because there is a larger surface to cover, it is well to stroke with alternate hands. . . . There should be about six alternate hand strokings over the posterior surface of the thigh. . . ."[6]

Others

McMillan uses both *simultaneous stroking* and *one-hand stroking*, but does not make reference to the use of knuckling, thumb stroking, or one hand over the other for deeper pressure.[7]

[4] *Ibid.*, pp. 36-38.

[5] *Ibid.*, p. 19.

[6] *Ibid.*, p. 25.

[7] McMillan, pp. 24, 26.

MC MILLAN'S PETRISSAGE TECHNIQUES

One- or Two-Hand Petrissage

"Petrissage or kneading may be performed either with the whole of the palmar surface of the hand or by fingers and thumb." [8]

Two-Finger Petrissage

"For picking up small muscles (as, for example, those of the face) the forefinger and thumb are use." [9]

Petrissage of the Back

For petrissage of the back she says, "Each section in turn is petrissaged by a pressure of muscles against the ribs, or, in the lumbar region, upon the abdominal wall. These muscles cannot be picked up as those in the limbs. The whole of the palmar surface of the hand is brought into play, but not in a molding manner as for the limbs, because the contour of the surface is flat instead of rounded." [10]

Alternate One-Hand Petrissage

"A useful variation of petrissage may be accomplished by the flexors and extensors being grasped by alternate hands, and a wringing movement being performed." [11]

Friction

Regarding friction McMillan says:

Friction, or circular friction, is that form of manipulation in which the tips of the fingers or the fingers and thumbs are used— more especially around the bony prominences of joint surfaces. Pressure in a circular manner is brought to bear upon the underlying structures. This form of manipulation is extremely useful in breaking down adhesions and in promoting absorption. Friction should be followed by effleurage in order to send on through the blood-stream the broken-down products of inflammation.

Friction is performed by circular movements with the finger-tips, or with two or three finger-tips, or even with one, according

---

[8] McMillan, p. 31.
[9] *Ibid.*
[10] *Ibid.*, pp. 33-34.
[11] *Ibid.*, p. 31.

to the amount of surface to be covered. . . . In friction of the phalangeal joints the joints of the first and third fingers are manipulated between the finger and thumb of the operator. In the same way the second and fourth fingers receive friction. . . .

Running frictions are sometimes used to advantage in a case of recovering sciatica. Over the denser area the thenar eminence is used for the circular frictions, starting over the great sciatic notch where the sciatic nerve emerges from the pelvis. These friction movements are carried down the whole area of the terminal endings of the sciatic nerve.[12]

McMillan, then, uses the *thumb, two or three fingers, or the thenar eminence* for friction.

Tapotement

Tapotement is a series of brisk blows, one following another in rapid succession. It may be performed in four ways: Hacking, clapping, tapping, and beating.

Hacking is the most common form of tapotement. The operator's hands are held with ulnar borders of each ready to strike. The fingers are slightly flexed and parted, and the hands strike alternately. As the blow falls the fingers strike together. They are then separated, and the hand is raised some distance from the patient before the blow is repeated. Hacking is performed so as to strike transversely across the muscle-fibers from one end of the muscle to the other. . . .

Clapping is done with a cupped hand, the fingers and thumb being slightly flexed and the palmar surface contracted. This form of tapotement is especially useful for covering the entire surface of the back. Clapping is also used over the chest muscles. It has a stimulating effect when used over peripheral vessels and nerves.

Tapping is performed with the fingers cone-shaped, and sharp, brisk tapping movements are applied with the tips to the surface desired. . . .

Beating is done with the ulnar border of the closed hand, as in making a fist. This form of tapotement is used over the gluteal muscles where the fascia is dense.[13]

Vibration

Vibration is performed with several fingers or even with one, and at times the whole palmar surface of the hand is used. A trembling sensation is conveyed by the operator. . . .[14]

[12] *Ibid.*, pp. 35-38.
[13] *Ibid.*, pp. 38-40.
[14] *Ibid.*, p. 41.

Massage of the Upper Extremity

In the first division of effleurage of the arm the palmar surface of the operator's hand supports the palmar surface of the patient's hand. The operator's working or active hand is then placed finger-tips to finger-tips with those of the patient; if the thumb-to-thumb method is adopted, it is much easier to fit hand to hand. Three or four firm, even strokings on the dorsal surface of the patient's hand are given. In order to conserve time and energy the operator, without changing hands, turns the patient's hand from the prone to the supine position; the supporting hand of the operator then becomes the active hand. The palmar surface is then stroked three or four times in a similar manner. In effleurage of the forearm the patient's hand is in the middle position between pronation and supination. One hand of the operator is used for the flexor group, while the other hand is supporting the part; then the hands should be reversed for the extensor group. The hands are now in position for effleurage of the upper arm, which is the third division. In a similar manner the flexor and extensor groups, each in turn, are stroked.[15]

McMillan then follows these same divisions, using petrissage and friction. She describes a useful variation of petrissage which may be used on both the flexors and the extensors. Grasping the flexors in one hand and the extensors in the other she performs an alternate wringing movement.[16]

Massage of the Lower Extremity

In discussing massage of the lower extremity McMillan states:

Subdivisions of the lower extremity correspond to those of the upper: First, foot; second, leg; third, thigh. In effleurage of the lower extremity the same procedure is used as with the upper extremity. The leg which is being massaged should never hang from the knee-joint, but should be well supported from the hip-joint.

The plantar surface of the foot from the tips of the toes to the heel is stroked with one hand. The other hand takes the stroke on the dorsal surface from the toes to beyond the ankle-joint. The whole palmar surface of the hand should conform to the sole of the foot.

The leg should be grasped with one hand covering the muscles on one side of the crest of the tibia, the other hand grasping the

[15] *Ibid.*, pp. 22-24.
[16] *Ibid.*, p. 31.

muscles on the other side. In this way one hand covers the anterior tibial group and the peroneal, while the other hand grasps the gastrocnemius group, the underlying and posterior tibial group being affected by the pressure from the superficial group. Always, where there are several layers of muscles, especially where the muscles are much developed, the stroking should be deeper, in order to reach the veins and lymphatic vessels which lie nearest the bone.

The third division of the lower extremity is the thigh. Here, because there is a larger surface to cover, it is well to stroke with alternate hands. At first both hands grasp the limb, finger-tips touching in the popliteal space, between inner and outer hamstring muscles. There should be about six alternate hand strokings over the posterior surface of the thigh, bringing the hands over the lateral aspects of the thigh to the anterior surface, where similar action is brought into play, until the whole of the thigh has been thoroughly stroked. This completes the general outline for effleurage of the limbs.[17]

McMillan then follows these same divisions using petrissage and friction. Concerning petrissage she states:

The lower extremity also is divided into three divisions. The foot is petrissaged, special attention being paid to the muscles of the plantar surface. The hand of the operator, making special use of the thenar eminence, kneads well into the plantar muscles. As the dorsum of the foot is so tendinous, petrissage is supplemented by running frictions between the interossei muscles. The spine of the tibia is used as a guide for the thumb of the operator in petrissage of the leg. On one side of the spine the muscles are kneaded by one hand, and on the other side of the spine by the other. If the small anterior tibial muscles require special care, finger-and-thumb petrissage is useful, as the muscle group is small and lies snugly against the tibia. In giving petrissage to the quadriceps group the two hands are used as one, the thumb of the right hand lying alongside the forefinger of the left hand, or vice versa. In this way the two hands, as one, pick up the anterior thigh muscles. The adductors and hamstrings are petrissaged by alternate hands.[18]

Massage of the Back

It is well to divide the back into four main divisions, as there is so great an extent of surface. The patient should be in prone

[17] *Ibid.*, pp. 24-26.

[18] *Ibid.*, pp. 32-33.

lying position on a straight plinth or bed with no pillows under the head. This position cannot be assumed by patients suffering from heart complication or from phthisis [tuberculosis] in which a hacking cough is aggravated by this position. In either of these cases, or when it is found inadvisable for the patient to lie flat, the back may be massaged while the patient is in a sitting posture. In general, however, the prone lying position is not at all uncomfortable for the majority of patients.

The first division of the back is from behind the ears, along the slope of the neck muscles, to the tip of the shoulder-girdle (Figure 21-1). At the beginning of the stroke the forefinger is separated from the other fingers in order to get well behind the ears, and the stroke is carried until all the fingers come in close contact with each other again at the nape of the neck. With the same firm, even pressure, the stroke is then carried to its termination at the acromion process. In this division both hands of the operator start below the inferior angle of the scapulae and work in opposite directions from the center line, the stroke being repeated several times.

In the third division the hands start over the region of the sacrum and both hands stroke upward on corresponding sides until they reach the axilla. They are then brought back, one on each side of the trunk, each describing a circular movement. Care should be taken to cover the whole area with the upward stroke.

The glutei is the last division of the back. Here heavier pressure should be exerted on account of the density of fascia in the region. The operator, starting with one hand on each side of the

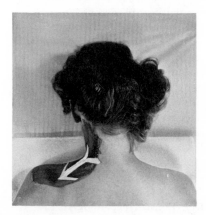

Figure 21-1. Upper trapezius, first division.

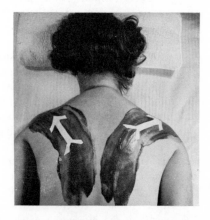

Figure 21-2. Middle and lower trapezius, second division. (Second division not discussed in McMillan's text, but shown in illustration, page 27.

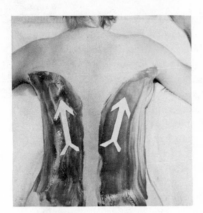

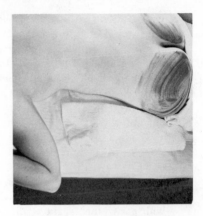

Figure 21-3. Latissimus dorsi, third divison.

Figure 21-4. Gluteals, fourth division.

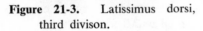

buttocks, strokes from the apex of the sacrum over the whole of the gluteal muscles, coming back without pressure to the starting-point. When each division of the back has been effleuraged, it is well to cover the whole surface with long, firm, even strokes from the sacrum to the nape of the neck.

The back is divided in the same way for petrissage as for effleurage. Each section in turn is petrissaged by a pressure of muscle against the ribs, or, in the lumbar region, upon the abdominal wall. (sic) These muscles cannot be picked up as those in the limbs. The whole of the palmar surface of the hand is brought into play, but not in a molding manner as for the limbs, because the contour of the surface is flat instead of rounded.

The glutei muscles and fascia, being dense, require a much deeper kneading than those in any other region. The kneading movement over the glutei is similar to that in kneading dough. . . . After effleurage, petrissage, and tapotement of the first and second divisions of the back are completed, those parts are covered to protect them. The third and fourth divisions receive the same treatment, except that the glutei region, being more dense, gets beating instead of hacking. The cover is now entirely removed and the final procedure of effleurage is enacted, four to six strokes being administered, and each stroke extending the whole distance from the sacrum to the acromion. Tapotement in the form of brisk tapping for its stimulating effect, or light rhythmical hacking for its sedative effect, is used, according to the needs of the individual patient. Cupping the muscles, the hands being used alternately and making longitudinal sweeps each side of the spinal column, contributes the final procedure for the back.[19]

[19] *Ibid.*, pp. 26-29, 33-34, 70.

SUMMARY

Mary McMillan's influence has spread throughout the United States, the Philippines, China, and Europe. Her dynamic personality carried her to far parts of the world, and wherever she went people could not help but feel her progressive influence. Through the army training schools her techniques for positioning of the patient, maintaining contact on the return stroke, stroking off the whole area, and alternate-hand effleurage and petrissage became an integral part of massage in the United States.

Chapter 22

James B. Mennell

Mennell says very little about the exact technique of massage except to describe the various strokes. He classifies these as: stroking, divided into superficial stroking and deep effleurage; and compression movements, divided into kneading, frictions, pressures, and petrissage. His terminology differs from common usage. He refers to friction as *frictions*, and divides petrissage into *kneading* and *petrissage*, the kneading referring to the circular, two-hand type of petrissage which is similar to McMillan's two-hand petrissage.

Most of the emphasis in his book is placed on a slow and even rhythm, a gentle and light pressure, and a longer term of instruction for the operator. A great deal of space is devoted to the physiological effects accomplished by massage rather than on the actual technique. According to Mennell, it is of maximum importance in massaging a given part to begin away from the part which is injured or diseased and work gradually toward it.

In reference to the patient's relaxation, Mennell states:

> The resistance offered by muscular contraction in the part under treatment to deep stroking is so great as to render it practically useless. As the first essential is to ensure that the whole part is in a state of perfect relaxation, careful attention must be given to the posture, not only of the part under treatment, but of the patient's whole body. If necessary, relaxation must be procured by preliminary superficial stroking. If the muscles are relaxed, they offer to the movement no more resistance than so much fluid, and therefore it is obvious that any pressure, exerted

on the surface, will be transmitted freely to all the structures under the hand. A pressure of 10 mm. of mercury will suffice to attain any objective desired by the use of the movement, except perhaps the mechanical emptying of a dilated lymphatic. A little practice, combined with a skill that is born only of a delicate sense of touch, will show how very light may be the pressure which will suffice to compress any structure to its full extent, and therefore, incidentally, to empty the veins and lymphatic spaces. Also there is no call for great rapidity of movement. The flow of blood in the veins is slow, and of the lymph in its channels still slower. There is no object in performing a movement to empty a vein if sufficient time has not elapsed for blood to flow into it, since the last movement ceased. Moreover, a heavy pressure, a very rapid movement, or even a jarring contact may convey to the patient the fear of a possible chance of injury, be the fear conscious or subconscious. A protective reflex may then be excited, the muscle may contract, and so the one condition under which we can perform our work to the greatest advantage is sacrificed. . . .

Unless contra-indications exist, we may take it for granted that deep stroking should commence over the proximal segment of a limb before we attack the distal, so as to ensure the "removal of the cork from the bottle." [1]

Regarding the patient's position, Mennell points out that the patient should be generally comfortable, with the head supported, abdominals and thigh muscles relaxed, and the feet supported. The operator should maintain a stance which is, in general, comfortable, with no strain on the back muscles or knees. The position should be such that one can reach the whole limb and support it properly.

MENNELL'S TECHNIQUES

Superficial Stroking

Since superficial stroking is a distinctive part of Mennell's massage techniques, its description is included here in its entirety.

Though it is possible to trace a reflex response to most of the movements of massage, this is the only movement which aims at securing no other effect.

The essentials to remember in using this treatment are that our movements must be slow, gentle, and rhythmical and yet they must be given with what one can only describe as a confident

[1] Mennell, *Physical Treatment by Movement, Manipulation, and Massage,* pp. 28-29.

touch; there must be no doubt, hesitancy or irregularity about it.

The slowness is important, as without it the other two essentials are impossible. If the stroke is to pass from hand to shoulder, some fifteen movements a minute will suffice. Moreover, the movement of the masseur's hand throughout must be continuous and even, not only while the hand is in contact with the part, but also during the return through the air, when there must be no contact. Occasionally we hear it stated that loss of contact between the hand and the part is conducive to a chilling of the patient. This can only be due to inefficient performance, when the movement may convey a "creepy" sensation. This is usually the outcome of timidity, or of lack of training and practice.

The call for gentleness is obvious, as we are avowedly attempting to secure no mechanical effect. The firmness of the pressure should be sufficient only to ensure that the patient is actually conscious of the passage of the hand throughout the entire movement. Thus there should be no question of the patient being able to detect the passage of the hand over a certain point during one movement, while being unable to note it during subsequent movements. Otherwise the sensation conveyed by one movement cannot be identical with that conveyed by each subsequent movement. Firmness is essential, but only the lightest possible pressure.

The need for rhythm can be readily understood, as without it the nature of the stimulus will be uneven, and the recation also will thereby be rendered uneven.

There should be no sensation of jarring at the beginning or end of the stroke, and the time that elapses between the end of one stroke and the commencement of the next must be identical throughout the whole of the treatment. To attain all these requisites it is essential to develop a "swing," and the portion of the "swing" which takes place while the hand is not in contact with the limb is as important as that during which hand and skin are in contact. Throughout the treatment the masseur's hand must remain supple, with all muscles relaxed, so that it may mould itself naturally to the contour of the limb, thus ensuring greater perfection of contact, and bringing as wide an area as possible under treatment. . . . If we wish to secure nothing but a reflex response to our movement, it may safely be left to the patient to decide the direction. If movement in one direction is more pleasing (i.e., more sedative) than another, there can be no objection to using it, even though the movement be centrifugal. Surface stroking "against the grain" of a hairy limb may be devoid of comfort, and, if so, it cannot be expected to call forth a beneficent reflex. It can only annoy. Shaving the part might be expected to help: it does not, and the process is not recommended save in the rarest of cases.

But whatever may be the direction chosen, one rule must be

strictly obeyed, namely, that the stroking is performed in the one direction only. Thus, if we are stroking the back of a patient suffering from insomnia, our stroke should be from cervical or thoracic region downwards, or to the cervical or thoracic region upwards, never from sacrum to thoracic region and then out over the shoulder with a downward tendency at the end. In the same way, if a leg is being stroked upwards, the utmost care must be taken not to allow the hand to come into contact with any part of the limb during the return; otherwise the stimulus will be broken and the reaction thereby rendered imperfect. This is in direct opposition to the advice of a former writer to "feather your oars" when using stroking movements. By this he meant that heavy centripetal stroking should be followed by light centrifugal stroking. . . .

. . . The most common mistake is to scratch the patient with the pads of the fingers towards the end of each stroke. The second common error is to ignore the necessity for controlling the return of the hand through the air, and so to make this part of the movement less rhythmical than the stroking itself. A third main fault in technique is to ignore the necessity of selecting one definite direction for the movement, and, once having made the selection, of keeping to it. Another point, and one that is often overlooked, is that not only the hand, but every joint in the limb must be perfectly relaxed and perfectly supple.[2]

Deep Effleurage

Mennell believes that this movement may be deep without being forcible, in any sense of the word. It is essential to ensure perfect relaxation (if necessary, this can be acquired through superficial stroking). A pressure of 10 mm of mercury will suffice to obtain any objective desired by the use of the movement, except perhaps the mechanical emptying of a dilated lymphatic. Since the flow of blood and lymph is slow, this stroke should not be rapidly executed.[3]

Others

Aside from using *both hands simultaneously,* or *one hand at a time* as the occasion demands, Mennell does not use any other effleurage strokes.

Mennell distinguishes between kneading and petrissage; therefore, his description of both will be included here.

[2] *Ibid.,* pp. 24-27.
[3] *Ibid.,* pp. 27-28.

Kneading

This is performed with the two hands placed on opposite sides of the limb, the whole of the palmar surface being in contact with the part. Gentle pressure is then exerted and a circular movement performed, the hands usually working in an opposite direction. Pressure is so regulated that it is not even throughout the movement, but should be greatest while the hand is engaged with the lowest part of the circumference of the circle, and least when at the opposite pole. This is effected by imparting a slight rotation to the wrist, the hand being more supinated below than above. The movement commences over the proximal portion of the limb; the pressure is then reapplied at the next most distal part and the movement repeated.[4]

Petrissage

The movement consists of grasping the muscle-mass between the fingers and thumbs of both hands and raising it away from the subjacent tissues. The tissues grasped are then compressed alternately between the thumb of one hand and the fingers of the other. The hands are made to slide away gently over the surface, until the whole region has been manipulated. Care should be taken to avoid an all-too-common error in technique: dragging the fingers over the surface. Instead of merely exerting an intermittent pressure, the grip should be soft and the whole hand relaxed (Figure 22-1). Sometimes when the muscular tissue is sufficiently bulky, each picking-up movement is made to alternate with a kneading movement.

> A third method, applicable chiefly to the calf, is performed by picking up the muscle in one or both hands and carrying it from side to side with an inclination to upward movement at the same time. The result is an almost semicircular movement. . . . Any movement that calls forth a protective contraction can only defeat our aims, and should be regarded as an error in technique.[5]

Friction

Regarding friction Mennell says:

> In using frictions the object in view is to press deeply on the part under treatment and then to move the hand in a more or

[4] *Ibid.*, p. 31.
[5] *Ibid.*, p. 39.

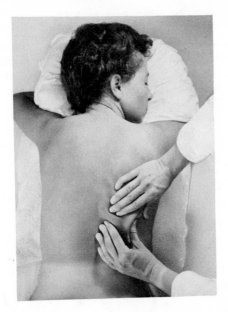

Figure 22-1. Mennell's petrissage to the back.

less circular direction. Any part of the hand may be used, but that generally employed is the tips of the fingers, or tip or ball of the thumb. . . .

Friction directed transversely to the long axis of muscle fibers will often aid in securing relaxation.[6]

Although he says that any part of the hand may be used, he recommends the use of the *tips of the fingers and the ball of the thumb.*

Mennell's use of the term "frictions" instead of "friction" should be noted since he feels quite strongly that all massage is in a sense "friction," and therefore attempts to distinguish the terms by using this terminology.

Tapotement

Mennell describes tapotement under the title of "percussion movements."

Hacking. This may be performed with the ulnar border of the little finger, either alone or supplemented in turn by the other fingers—the result being a series of soft blows, the first from the

[6] *Ibid.,* pp. 33-34.

little finger direct, the others from each successive finger in turn transmitted through the finger or fingers that have already delivered their tap. Sometimes the little finger is curled up in the palm of the hand, and only the middle fingers are used. If a more vigorous action is deemed necessary, the ulnar surface of the whole hand may be used with all the fingers kept close together and partially flexed but not rigid. The tips or palmar surfaces of the three middle fingers can be used. . . .

Clapping. The hands are so held that the fingers and palm form a concave arch, and in this position they are brought sharply into contact with the body. The result is a rather deep-toned clapping sound. . . .

Beating. This is the most vigorous form of percussion massage. The fist is half closed, and either the ulnar or the palmar surface is used for beating the surface of the body. If no force is put into the movement, it may be used over bony areas such as the sacrum and over areas well covered by muscle, such as the gluteal region. As our only hope from its use in these regions is to secure a reflex action it should be performed lightly.[7]

Vibration

Regarding vibration Mennell says:

Hand vibration is a poor substitute for many of the mechanical vibrators on the market. . . . It is true that a few—a very few— masseurs have been able to develop a technique of administering vibration with their hands to such a degree of proficency that manual treatment is preferable to that derived from apparatus.[8]

SUMMARY

Mennell's theory of "uncorking the bottle" by massaging the proximal aspect of the limb before the distal is now being practiced by most people. As a rule they are following his principle of adapting the treatment to the individual patient's needs, rather than treating by a specific routine which concerns number of strokes or length of treatment. His influence has been widely felt throughout the United States and Europe. His constant emphasis is on the gentle approach, beginning away from the sensitive part and working slowly toward it. His use of massage, combined with careful, relaxing, passive movement, is very effective.

[7] *Ibid.*, pp. 40-41.

[8] *Ibid.*, p. 44.

Supplemental Learning and Teaching Materials

Chapter 23

Cases for Analysis and Planning of Treatment Program

Regardless of the injury or illness of the patient, the operator will be dealing with such conditions as pain, swelling, scar tissue, muscle spasm, fibrositic nodules, muscle splinting, poor skin condition following casting, contractures, and insufficiencies of circulation. Students of massage should be exposed to other courses such as pathology, orthopedics, surgery, and neurology, in order to understand the injuries and illnesses they will be dealing with. The following lists of indications and contraindications will give an overview of situations commonly treated by massage and those for which massage might do more harm than good.

Indications

Each indication should be considered with the view that there are times when it might *not* profit by massage. No one can be expected to do an adequate job of massage without a thorough understanding of the medical implications of each situation. If a certain effect is desired, the operator must determine how it can be obtained.

In most of the following situations, massage would be indicated during a subacute phase *but not during an acute phase:*

Amputations	Myositis
Arthritis	Neurasthenia
Burns	Orthopedic and neurological
Bursitis	situations
Contractures	Peripheral neuritis
Decubitus areas, and surrounding tissue	Poliomyelitis
	Postural deviations
Facial paralysis (Bell's palsy)	Scar tissue (certain adhesions)
	Strains and sprains
Fractures	Tension headache
Insomnia	Torticolis
Long bed rest	

Contraindications

Massage should be used in the following conditions only under the most careful medical guidance, never by a new student unless most carefully supervised, and always with utmost caution.

Cardiac decompensation

Edema, obstructive or decompensated, also inflammatory or noninfectious

Hematomas

Herniated disc

Mental states, particularly depressive or manic

Nonunion fractures

Phlebitis

Postoperative

    tendon transplants

    orthopedic cases

    neurological cases

Severe lacerations

Spastic paralyses, such as: Parkinson's, multiple sclerosis, hemiplegias, paraplegias, congenital cerebral palsies, traumatic or post-surgical brain injuries, encephalitis

In many situations, the consequences of massage would be obvious to the operator, who understands its physiological or mechanical effects. One must be aware of the damage that can be done by the indiscriminate use of massage.

Any of the conditions listed under indications that appear acute should be considered as contraindicated for massage. In addition, one should be sure that none of the following conditions exists before proceeding with massage.

Abdominal massage is contraindicated in the event of pregnancy, large
  hernias, or any possibility of peritonitis or appendicitis

Acute tubercular lesions, malignancies

Cellulitis

Certain neurotic conditions, especially emotional instabilities

Debilitating diseases

Edema due to heart decompensation or kidney ailments, synovitis,
  thrombus which may be dislodged, embolism, sinusitis

Fever

Massage that aggravates the patient's mental or physical condition

Localized acute infections

New surgery

Skin eruptions that may exacerbate

Undiagnosed friends

CASES FOR ANALYSIS AND PLANNING
OF TREATMENT PROGRAM

The following cases include the diagnosis and treatment prescribed. They have been designed for the purpose of helping students see the relationship between disabilities and the planning that is needed to organize the massage treatment. By thinking these cases through, one can relate theory and practice. Greater confidence will be developed, professional attitudes will be strengthened, and effective reasoning and problem-solving ability will improve. The organization of a case will increase understanding of the disorder.

Names, dates, record numbers, addresses, number and frequency of treatments, doctor's signatures, and dates for re-examination by the doctor have been deliberately ignored in writing the following cases. This is to focus attention on the massage. Such information is usually included in case reports, but here it would only be repetitive.

These cases include situations that involve many parts of the body and encompass conditions which are often treated by massage.

Users of this text who do not have adequate background or supplementary courses in anatomy, physiology and pathology, or are not taking a course with a qualified instructor who can competently guide and correct their plans, will profit little by this approach and should not attempt to analyze these cases by themselves. *In some instances these cases deliberately include situations which should not be massaged at all.* In these cases students should know why massage would not be advisable. *In other cases inadequate or inaccurate information is provided.* In such cases people should realize this and be able to state what questions need to be answered before treatment can be given. *In several instances the treatment ordered is incorrect.* In these cases people should seek accurate treatment instructions, or be ready to recommend more appropriate treatments.

The following outline will assist in the study of these cases. With the guidance and assistance of a qualified instructor, one can become more aware of the many things that have to be considered whenever a brief diagnosis is given. In each case one should seek the following information:

1. Adequate description of the injury or illness.

2. Significant dates of onset, surgery, casts, etc.

3. Necessary supportive measures: braces, crutches, and support needed during treatment.

4. Treatment requested (is it adequate? accurate?).

5. Precautions, indications and contraindications for the treatment requested.

In preparing to massage these cases one should consider:

1. Purposes of the treatment, such as reduction of swelling, increase in range of motion, reduction of pain, relaxation, etc.

2. Creation of relaxed environment, establishment of good social and professional relationship.

3. Additional information that might be needed.

4. Positioning and draping to be used.

5. Assistance with dressing and undressing.

6. Choice and use of lubricant, if any.

7. Organization of the massage treatment to include:
   a. Efficient use of time and equipment.
   b. Area to be treated.
   c. Direction, rhythm, and choice of treatment to be given.
   d. Pressure to be used, tolerance of patient to pressure.
   e. Body mechanics of the operator.
   f. Termination of treatment, equipment to replace, cleaning of treatment table, arrangements for next appointment, etc.
   g. Other types of treatment to be given in addition to massage.

8. Evaluation of effectiveness of treatment. (What observations can be made that will indicate whether or not the objectives of treatment have been accomplished?)

SAMPLE CASE

The following case has been analyzed for use as a sample.

Information Provided for the Operator

Diagnosis: A three-year-old boy has received a severe burn to the right wrist. There is extensive scar tissue and flexion contractures at the wrist joint.

Treatment: Massage to the right forearm and hand, in preparation for stretching.

Analysis as Done By the Operator:

Description of Injury: The description does not tell how the boy was burned nor when, how extensively the wrist is involved except that it was extensive enough to leave a scar and cause contractures at the wrist. Some of this information could be quickly learned by examining the patient. Usually it is helpful to know how the accident happened. Such information could be obtained from the person requesting the treatment or the patient's chart.

Significant Dates: There is no indication of the date of the accident. This could probably be found by checking the patient's chart.

Support: No support should be needed other than for the comfort of the patient.

Treatment Requested: There is no request for heat preceding massage, nor for stretching of the contractures. One may suggest the importance of combining stretching with massage to regain normal motion. One should also initiate an exercise program.

Precautions: Be assured that the scar tissue is strong enough to permit this type of treatment and seek further information as to the extent of the deep scar tissue. Review the pathology of burns.[1]

Purpose of Treatment: The purpose of massage in this case would be to promote relaxation, stretch tissue, encourage active motion, improve local blood supply, and increase range of motion.

Gaining Confidence: At the onset of treatment, gaining this little boy's confidence will be more important than the amount of motion regained. The approach should be friendly and gentle, causing no undue pain. When he is fully aware of the objectives of his treatment program he can then be asked to cooperate, even to the extent of enduring any necessary pain. Find out what he likes to do with his hands and encourage him to try to do all he can for himself.

Additional Information Needed

One needs to know the depth of the burn, how it happened, whether the elbow flexors are also tight, whether the finger flexors are involved, and the condition of the scar tissue.

Position

Since the patient is three years old he would probably be comfortable sitting on a treatment table with a pillow in his lap. This would put him high enough to work with easily. He might also be comfortable lying down on the treatment table, letting his arm rest on it.

Draping

Remove his shirt. Leave the undershirt on if it has no sleeves. Put a towel about the shoulders.

Assistance with dressing

Let the parents help him until he is acquainted with the operator.

Lubricant
Use cocoa butter which is thought to be good for scar tissue.

---

[1] See W. A. D. Anderson, *Pathology*, 3rd ed. (St. Louis: The C. V. Mosby Co., 1957). First, second and third degree burns, pp. 133-34.

Organization of Treatment

Time: Allow time to get acquainted for the first treatment; possibly 30 minutes, later massage could probably be done in about 15 minutes.

Area to be Treated: If the elbow is also tight from protective positioning, the entire arm should be included in the massage. The upper arm and elbow should be massaged before concentrated work on the wrist and hand is done.

Choice of Technique: Treatment of the upper extremity would be done as described in Chapter 13 of this text. In addition to this, deep effleurage strokes which stretch while they stroke should be carried out. By working into these strokes gradually the patient will tolerate greater stretching. Stretching should never exceed the pain tolerance of the patient and should begin and end gradually. If there is no swelling, stretching strokes may pull downward against the venous flow. These should be followed by effleurage strokes which go with the venous flow. Keeping in mind that massage cannot break up deep adhesions or scar tissue, active motion should be encouraged. Much of the tightness present may be due to protective muscle splinting against pain. If this is so, good results can be expected. Treatment should be concluded with effleurage to the entire arm, working from deep pressure to light.

Pressure: Pressure should stay well within the pain tolerance of the patient.

Body mechanics of the operator: Body mechanics of the operator should be no problem with the patient on the treatment table.

Termination of treatment: Every effort should be made to finish treatment with the patient in good spirits and enthusiastic about returning for further treatment. Attention to him should take preference over straightening-up activities that can be done when he has left.

Other types of treatment: Although the prescription only calls for massage, combined stretching and active exercise should be included. This boy could also profit from occupational therapy to encourage functional reeducation for the entire arm and hand.

How to Tell if Objectives Have Been Accomplished

If range of motion increases (determined by goniometer measurements compared with the first day of treatment), the major objective of treatment has been accomplished. If the boy relaxes and cooperates with the program, treatment will be more effective. If the functional use of the boy's arm continues to improve, it can be assumed that treatment is accomplishing the objectives for which it was designed. If no increase in range of motion is noticeable, he should be referred for other treatment approaches or to a different operator.

Summary

This is an example illustrating how cases may be analyzed and treated. Each person may think of different ways to deal with every case. Regardless of how it is done, the experience of working out programs for oneself is where the real value of this exercise lies.

CASE 1

Diagnosis

A three-year-old boy has received a severe burn to the right wrist. There is extensive scar tissue and flexion contractures at the wrist joint.

Treatment

Massage to the right forearm and hand in preparation for stretching.

CASE 2

Diagnosis

A 50-year-old woman has hypertension and is unable to sleep.

Treatment

Back massage to encourage relaxation.

CASE 3

Diagnosis

A 20-year-old male's right shoulder and arm have just been removed from a cast after surgery to relieve recurrent shoulder dislocation.

Treatment

Give tapotement, effleurage, and petrissage to deltoid and trapezius in an attempt to increase circulation and relieve spasm.

CASE 4

Diagnosis

A railroad worker lost his left foot when he fell beneath a train six weeks ago. Surgical repair has been done and a stump seven inches below the knee remains. There are flexion contractures at the knee.

Treatment

Give massage to the left leg, including gentle to increasing percussion to the stump end.

CASE 5

Diagnosis

A 55-year-old taxi driver has had severe bursitis in the right shoulder for two years.

Treatment

Give heat, massage, and exercise to the right shoulder.

CASE 6

Diagnosis

A football player suffered a torn semilunar cartilage in last week's game. The knee is swollen and tender. He cannot bear weight on it.

Treatment

Very light massage to reduce spasm and pain.

CASE 7

Diagnosis

A 43-year-old woman suffered amputation of the left breast two weeks ago due to a malignant tumor. The shoulder is painful and motion is limited.

Treatment

Massage to relieve pain and increase motion.

CASE 8

Diagnosis

A truck driver crushed his foot, receiving multiple fractures, eight weeks ago. The foot is swollen and painful. Motion at the ankle joint is limited. Recent X rays show all fractures have healed.

Treatment

Massage to reduce swelling, reduce pain, and increase motion of all joints involved. Preheat the part by using whirlpool at 110° F and follow massage with exercise.

CASE 9

Diagnosis

A paraplegic woman has developed a large decubitus ulcer over the sacrum.

Treatment

Massage surrounding tissues to stimulate circulation.

CASE 10

Diagnosis

A 15-year-old girl was in an automobile accident. She has a fractured right femur which confines her to bed, in traction. In addition to the femur there are fractures to the jaw and left elbow. She complains of severe pain in the back due to the uncomfortable position caused by traction to the leg.

Treatment

Give massage to the back. Please move this patient as little as possible.

CASE 11

Diagnosis

Onset of polio was diagnosed 10 days ago in a 10-year-old boy. He has severe spasm of the hamstrings of both legs.

Treatment

Hot pack and massage both lower extremities.

CASE 12

Diagnosis

A 40-year-old professor has severe low back pain from a herniated disc with severe sciatica associated. Any right leg movements which stretch the sciatic nerve are painful.

Treatment

Give petrissage to the low back.

CASE 13

Diagnosis

A boy received a greenstick fracture of the right ulna two weeks ago. The cast was removed two days ago.

Treatment

Give massage to the right arm.

CASE 14

Diagnosis

A patient was operated on for a herniated disc at the fourth cervical level one week ago. There is slight swelling in the area.

Treatment

Massage, attempting to reduce swelling and relieve associated muscle spasm.

CASE 15

Diagnosis

A 35-year-old woman received a fracture of the right humerus six weeks ago. The cast has been removed. There is limitation of motion at the shoulder and the elbow. The skin is irritated and tender. Heat has been applied.

Treatment

Massage in preparation for passive motion of the arm and shoulder.

CASE 16
Diagnosis

A 43-year-old woman has a suspected tumor at the C-3 level.

Treatment

Give deep massage, both petrissage and tapotement.

CASE 17
Diagnosis

A 45-year-old laborer suffers with myositis of the right upper trapezius.

Treatment

Give heat and massage to relieve pain and relax spasm.

CASE 18
Diagnosis

A neuropsychiatric patient is 25 years old and in a manic depressive state.

Treatment

Give back massage for sedation.

CASE 19
Diagnosis

A patient has had severe arthritis of the whole body for the past 15 years. There is marked limitation of motion in the left knee; no motion of the patella; and a flexion deformity of the knee at 145°.

Treatment

Give massage to mobilize the left knee.

CASE 20

Diagnosis

The cast has just been removed from a well-healed fracture of the right elbow of an eight-year-old boy.

Treatment

Massage and exercise to mobilize the joint and strengthen the muscles.

CASE 21

Diagnosis

A female, age 57, fell and dislocated her left shoulder four weeks ago. She carries her arm in an airplane splint. There is also a stretch injury to the brachial plexus.

Treatment

Massage the entire shoulder, arm, and hand, being careful not to change the position of the shoulder.

CASE 22

Diagnosis

A 30-year-old concert pianist suffers from chronic tenosynovitis of the middle finger of the left hand.

Treatment

Give paraffin bath to be followed by massage.

CASE 23

Diagnosis

A college basketball player sprained his ankle yesterday. There is considerable swelling; much pain exists.

Treatment

Massage in attempt to decrease swelling and get this player back into the game as soon as possible.

CASE 24

Diagnosis

A boy's elbow was hyperextended when he fell while ice skating, causing some tearing of the ligaments. Extension to 150° elicits pain. There is slight swelling and discoloration; the elbow is still tender.

Treatment

Heat has been applied. Massage in an attempt to reduce swelling and alleviate pain.

CASE 25

Diagnosis

A young female patient has had acute myositis of the left tibialis anterior since an automobile accident about a year ago. There remains an area of "hardness" in the midshin region which limits the contracting range of the muscle.

Treatment

Massage to increase range of motion of the ankle joint.

CASE 26

Diagnosis

A 50-year-old bricklayer has a chronic low back pain from an old lumbosacral strain.

Treatment

Massage.

CASE 27

Diagnosis

A 50-year-old man has Bell's palsy on the right side following surgery for removal of a nonmalignant tumor of the parotid gland.

Treatment

Massage.

CASE 28

Diagnosis

A professor has been having tension headaches involving spasm of the muscles of the upper back and neck, especially on the right side.

Treatment

Massage to relieve tension in upper back and neck.

CASE 29

Diagnosis

An 18-year-old boy has a "baseball finger," the index finger of the right hand, with a chip fracture of the metacarpophalangeal joint. There is pain and swelling.

Treatment

Give heat, massage, and active exercise.

CASE 30

Diagnosis

A gunshot wound was received when this thirty-year-old man was cleaning his rifle. A .22 caliber bullet entered the body just below the right clavicle and emerged through the right scapula, shattering that bone and piercing the brachial plexus. The patient was injured six months ago and there has been no return of innervation from the damaged peripheral nerves. He carries his arm close to his body in a sling and complains of pain throughout the entire shoulder and arm.

Treatment

Give heat, and massage prior to faradic muscle testing.

CASE 31

Diagnosis

A 25-year-old butcher cut his arm just below the right elbow. The ulnar nerve injury had surgical repair two weeks ago.

Treatment

Give massage to the right lower arm and hand to increase circulation. Caution! Do not extend the elbow.

CASE 32

Diagnosis

A 60-year-old man has had arthritis of the spine. He stands in a slightly flexed position. Extension to normal standing position produces pain.

Treatment

Heat and massage to relieve pain and spasm.

CASE 33

Diagnosis

A 25-year-old secretary has a cervical rib which causes peripheral neuritis of the right upper extremity.

Treatment

Massage to relieve pain.

CASE 34

Diagnosis

A 16-year-old girl has a fracture of the neck of the right humerus following an automobile accident. She has been out of the cast for two days. There is little range of motion of the shoulder, elbow, wrist, or hand. There is swelling and pain.

Treatment

Massage in preparation for mobilization.

CASE 35

Diagnosis

A normal 20-year-old male is a star member of his college football team. Whether his team can win tomorrow will depend a great deal on how fast he can run and how far he can kick.

Treatment

Massage to precondition the player for peak performance the following day.

CASE 36

Diagnosis

Casting has just been removed from a four-year-old girl to correct bilaterally, congenitally dislocated hips.

Treatment

Use whirlpool followed by massage.

CASE 37

Diagnosis

A 10-year-old girl fell on the way home from the grocery store, breaking a bottle of milk and severely cutting the thenar eminence of her right hand on the broken fragments of glass. Tendon repair was done ten days ago.

Treatment

Very cautiously massage, precede with heat, and follow with gentle active exercise.

CASE 38

Diagnosis

A press-punch operator has developed a severe subdeltoid bursitis which inhibits his capacity to work.

Treatment

Use ultrasound, massage and exercise.

CASE 39

Diagnosis

A woman slipped going downstairs into the subway station, fracturing the posterior aspect of the right calcaneus, four weeks ago. She is suing the subway for injuries received, which may be the factor accounting for her seeming reluctance to regain normal range of motion.

Treatment

Give massage and exercise.

CASE 40

Diagnosis

A young woman fell from a horse three weeks ago. She was wearing glasses with metal frames. As she was dragged, with one foot caught in the stirrup, her face was deeply cut, tearing it from the lateral aspect of the right eye toward the mouth. The formation of keloid causes more disfiguration than normal and some adhesions are beginning to develop.

Treatment

Massage to loosen peripheral, adhesive scar tissue. If keloid formation increases refer her to a plastic surgeon for further treatment.

CASE 41

Diagnosis

A patient is just recovering from surgical treatment for Parkinson's disease on the right. The right hand is now free of spasm or tremor, but is stiff from disuse. The finger flexors remain tight, and the patient seems reluctant to try using his hand for daily activities.

Treatment

Give heat, massage, and exercise to assist the patient in regaining use of the hand.

CASE 42

Diagnosis

A patient has hysterical paralysis of both lower extremities following real, but nonparalytic polio. His younger sister suffers from paralysis of both lower extremities following polio just previous to the onset of her brother's.

Treatment

Give heat, massage, and exercise to support psychotherapy. This patient is to be approached exactly as if his paralysis were real. Any sign of muscle reeducation should be enthusiastically encouraged.

CASE 43

Diagnosis

A 21-year-old man had a triple arthrodesis four weeks ago for correction of a club foot.

Treatment

Massage in preparation for mobilization of foot.

CASE 44

Diagnosis

An 85-year-old woman had a total replacement of the right hip one week ago, following a nonunion fracture of the head of the femur.

Treatment

Give heat, massage, and exercise to the right hip.

CASE 45

Diagnosis

All fingers of the left hand of a 27-year-old housewife were crushed in the car door of the family station wagon. There were multiple fractures of all fingers across the tips, with some chip fractures into the first joint. The nail of the middle finger is off and those of the others in various stages of recovery.

Treatment

Massage the left hand, especially the fingers, in preparation for exercise to regain normal function of the hand.

In areas where one is able to work with patients early in his specialized education, cases that he is treating can be written up. The following outline [2] may be used:

A. Case History (to include the following):
   1. Present date.
   2. Age and sex of patient.
   3. Diagnosis and pathology (also contributing factors or complications, if any).
   4. Significant dates (onset, surgery, casts, etc.).
   5. Type of patient (wheel chair, crutches, ambulatory, etc.; distinguish between hospitalized and out-patients).

[2] This outline was created by Vera Kaska, Instructor of Massage, University of Connecticut School of Physical Therapy. It is reproduced here with her permission.

B. Treatment ordered (mention all treatment ordered but elaborate only on massage)
1. Type of treatment
2. Frequency of treatment

C. Precautions

D. Positioning
1. General position (sitting, lying supine, prone, etc.)
2. Support indicated (pillows, etc.)
3. Is elevation indicated?

E. Draping

F. Type of lubrication

G. Organization of routine (including amount of pressure used)

H. Duration of entire massage treatment (indicate approximately how time would be proportioned)

I. Termination

J. Source of information for history and treatment

SUMMARY

No one student can do justice in analysis of all these cases. Some can be assigned, while others can be used for group discussion. Others can be used in laboratory practice sessions. Any use made of them will increase the ability of people to meet and solve problems similar to those they will soon be facing. Any or all of the techniques discussed in this text should be considered when planning a treatment program.

Review Questions

These questions are designed to help people who wish to review this material for qualifying examinations.

1. Define massage.

2. On what basis would you judge treatment time for various patients?

3. Outline the important factors of personal appearance and cleanliness.

4. What postural considerations are important to the operator?

5. Name ten ways to assure comfort for the patient.

6. Name four fundamental facts pertaining to proper positioning of patients.

7. Outline the basic principles for draping a patient.

8. List the deciding factors in choice of lubricant or the use of none.

9. Name six lubricants and tell when you might use each.

10. Describe effleurage.

11. Diagram draping and positioning for massage of the back.

12. When the patient is lying prone, what consideration should be given to the position of the arms?

13. Describe all variations of effleurage.

14. Define the usefulness of petrissage.

15. List ten desirable qualities of personality of the operator.

16. Describe draping of the lower extremity, face-lying.

17. Briefly explain the place each name has in the history of massage and rearrange the names chronologically.

    a. Ambroise Paré
    b. Harving Nissen
    c. Albert Hoffa
    d. J. M. M. Lucas-Championnière
    e. Mary McMillan
    f. Hwang Ti
    g. Hippocrates
    h. Per Henrik Ling
    i. Gertrude Beard
    j. Homer
    k. James B. Mennell
    l. Elisabeth Dicke
    m. Sir William Bennett

18. How can you judge how much lubricant to use?

19. How does Storms' technique vary from the usual type of friction?

20. Would you ever give massage for skin nutrition only?

21. What is the effect of massage on sensory nerve endings?

22. How would you know when it is safe to massage scar tissue following burns?

23. What would massage do to affect normal function of the skin?

24. What is meant by reflex effects?

25. List the mechanical effects of massage.

26. Why should massage be done slowly if the objective is to assist the lymphatic flow?

27. Why is it important to rid the muscle of stagnant by-products of fatigue?

28. Explain how muscles normally maintain a metabolic balance.

29. Why is massage useful following overactivity?

30. Describe the metabolic picture following underactivity.

31. What is meant by venostasis?

32. Name three instances when you would *not* massage situations showing venostasis.

33. Name and explain four causes of edema.

34. Why does swelling occur in dependent limbs when normal activity has been limited?

35. Will massage be useful in eliminating edema in limbs suffering from extreme activity?

36. Why is massage not recommended in cases where edema is the result of recent injury?

37. Why is research in massage so difficult?

38. Will massage reduce obesity?

39. Of what use is massage following peripheral nerve injuries?

40. Does massage affect total blood flow?

41. Is massage more effective than electrical stimulation or passive exercise in increasing the flow of lymph?

42. Can massage ever adequately substitute for active exercise?

43. Describe massage as done by Cyriax.

44. Name five of the most used acupuncture points and list disabilities which could be relieved by finger pressure at these points, or combinations of these points.

45. Differentiate between Shiatsu and Oriental massage.

46. Discuss the possible mechanisms for relief of pain by massage or therapeutic touch.

47. List five areas on the foot where finger pressure (reflexology) could relieve symptoms in specific areas of the human body.

48. Discuss the importance of concern and empathy for a person while giving any kind of treatment that involves touching.

Appendix 1

Summary Chart
of Comparative Techniques

The following summary chart shows the results of a questionnaire determining the amount of use generally given to the various massage techniques. Twenty-five graduate operators were interviewed from fifteen different schools. These schools were: D.T. Watson School of Physical Therapy (Leetsdale, Pennsylvania); Children's Hospital (Los Angeles, California); Harvard University, Medical School, Courses for Graduates (Boston, Massachusetts); University of Southern California (Los Angeles, California); Mayo Clinic (Rochester, Minnesota); University of Minnesota (Minneapolis, Minnesota); Northwestern University, Medical School (Chicago, Illinois); New York University, School of Education (New York City); Stanford University (Stanford, California); University of Wisconsin, Medical School (Madison, Wisconsin); Reed College * (Portland, Oregon); Fitzsimmons General Hospital * (Denver, Colorado); O'Reilly General Hospital * (Springfield, Missouri); Walter Reed General Hospital * (Washington, D.C.); and The Institute of Southern Sweden (Stockholm, Sweden).

In order to prevent any one school from influencing the results, not more than three from each school were interviewed. In some instances, where the operator was teaching in one school but a graduate of another, it was considered that the information gathered was representative of the school in which that person was now teaching.

* Army Training Schools.

239

Question	Hoffa	McMillan	Mennell	Conclusions from Questionnaire Results
1. Are there any exceptions to following the venous flow?	The only exception is in the massage of the back, where the stroke may go in either direction.	No exceptions are made.	Exceptions include superficial stroking and following the principle of beginning away from the injured area.	The trend seems to be progressively toward making exceptions to following the venous flow as Mennell does.
2. What do you consider adequate treatment time for the back, a limb, and total body?	Six to ten minutes is used for back or limb and fifteen minutes for whole body.	Ten to fifteen minutes is recommended for beginners to use for the back or limb and not more than fifty minutes for a general massage.	Treatment time must depend on the pathology and reaction of the patient. No time can be suggested.	Treatment time must be adjustable to the pathology and reactions of the patient, but average between ten to twenty minutes for back or limb and up to forty-five for the whole body, which is more than Hoffa recommends and similar to McMillan's suggested time.
3. What do you prefer as a medium?	Anything to make the part pliable can be used.	Dry rubbing is preferred but for certain pathologies oil, cocoa butter or lanolin is suggested.	Mennell's prescription combines oil of Bergamot and French chalk.	Except in cases where pathology demands one or the other, choice of medium is up to the therapist, as Hoffa suggests.

The first column of the chart gives the questions asked; the second, third, and fourth columns explain, in brief, the methods of Hoffa, McMillan, and Mennell; and the last column gives the conclusions derived from the questionnaire results.

QUESTION	HOFFA	McMILLAN	MENNELL	CONCLUSIONS FROM QUESTIONNAIRE RESULTS
4. Do you massage by muscle groups or is massage done by other anatomical divisions of the body?	All massage is done by dividing the body into various muscle groups.	Some areas are divided by muscle groups and others, such as the back, are described using other anatomical landmarks.	Only the fact that one begins away from the injured part and works toward it, is mentioned as to how the area is covered.	The majority of operators still divide the body into specific muscle groups for massage as Hoffa does.
5. Is the most proximal part of the limb massaged before the distal?	Every description of a part to be massaged progresses from the distal aspect of the limb to the proximal.	Descriptions progress from the distal aspect of the limb to the proximal.	The proximal aspect of a limb should always be massaged before the more distal.	The practice of massaging the most proximal aspect of a limb before the distal as Mennell recommends is now being widely used.
6. Is the whole extremity or back effleuraged before petrissage is begun?	Each muscle or muscle group is given effleurage and petrissage before the next group is begun.	Massage of the leg is done by giving effleurage to the whole lower leg and then petrissage.	No definite routine in this respect is stated.	Most operators are still following the technique of massaging each muscle or muscle group with effleurage and petrissage before going to the next group as Hoffa does, rather than effleuraging a whole part and then giving it petrissage.

Question	Hoffa	McMillan	Mennell	Conclusions from Questionnaire Results
7. Is the patient always placed in a recumbent position?	The only time that the patient is in a recumbent position is in massage of the back, and even here the patient may be in a seated position.	The patient is always in a recumbent position unless pathology is such that this position cannot be held comfortably.	The patient is preferred in a recumbent position, but each patient must be considered individually. Thus sitting, or even standing positions may be used if necessary.	Most massage to the upper extremity is done with the patient in a seated position. The tendency seems to be that of making exceptions to the recumbent position as Mennell does.
8. Which parts are usually supported, (1) in a back-lying position, and (2) in a face-lying position?	(1) No back-lying position is described. (2) No mention of support is made with reference to the face-lying position.	(1) A rolled towel is placed under the knee. (2) A small pillow is placed under the abdomen.	(1) Support is placed under the knee. (2) The body is supported in slight hyperextension for back massage, with one pillow under the legs and another under the chest.	(1) Knees are supported in the back-lying position as by McMillan and Mennell. (2) Most people follow the technique of McMillan and support the abdomen, and all but three support the ankles or have them over the edge of the plinth.

242

QUESTION	HOFFA	McMILLAN	MENNELL	CONCLUSIONS FROM QUESTIONNAIRE RESULTS
9. What arm position is preferred when the patient is face-lying?	The arms are "out horizontally."	Arms are shown in "T" position and also down at the sides.	Arms are folded over the head. (Chest is supported by a pillow which relieves weight on the arms.)	McMillan's two positions are the ones used the most ("T" and at the sides), but the patient's comfort and ability to relax is the primary guide for selection of arm position.
10. In massage of the lower extremity is the patient usually turned from back-lying to face-lying?	The patient is turned to make the posterior thigh more accessible and is placed on the side to massage the tensor fascia lata.	The patient is not usually turned, but may be if pathological conditions are such that it seems best to do so.	The patient is turned to make the posterior thigh more accessible.	McMillan's policy of not turning the patient unless pathology indicates its necessity seems to be followed.
11. Must the part being massaged always be in elevation?	Hoffa seems to prefer a neutral position.	All illustrations show the part in a neutral position.	Elevation is preferred whenever possible.	Following Hoffa and McMillan, the trend is still that of elevating the part for pathological conditions and treating it otherwise in a neutral position.

243

Question	Hoffa	McMillan	Mennell	Conclusions from Questionnaire Results
12. Is emphasis placed on stance of the therapist?	No reference is made to stance.	No reference is made to stance.	Mennell mentions the operator should stand at the side of the table and not at the end. One should be comfortable, with no strain on the back or knees.	Little emphasis other than good body mechanics is placed on stance by everyone.
13. Do you alternate sides of the table during massage of the back?	The operator is instructed to move to the opposite side of the back when doing the other side.	No reference is made as to alternating sides of the table in massage of the back.	Mennell does alternate sides of the table during a back massage.	McMillan and the majority of the operators do not alternate sides of the table during massage of the back.
14. Do you always massage in a standing position?	Most of the massage is done with the operator seated, even in giving a massage to the back.	All illustrations show the operator in a standing position.	It is advised that all massage be done in a standing position.	Whereas people do not remain seated to the extent that Hoffa did, neither do they stand without exception. Hands and forearms are usually done with the operator seated.

Question	Hoffa	McMillan	Mennell	Conclusions from Questionnaire Results
15. Do you usually repeat a given stroke any particular number of times before progressing to a different stroke?	Hoffa refers to repeating a stroke "three or four" times but sets up no definite routine.	Suggestions for "three or four" strokes are included in descriptions. The number of strokes vary up to six and no set number is recommended.	Mennell makes no reference to number of strokes to be given.	The trend seems away from grouping strokes by numbers as indicated by the lack of mention of such in Mennell's text, and the fact that the majority of the people interviewed do not do so, except as a guide for beginners, which may have been all the basic texts meant it for.
16. Does return stroke always maintain contact?	Hoffa seems not to maintain contact with his return stroke.	The hand should return to its original position without pressure but without losing contact with the part being massaged.	The return stroke does not always maintain contact with the body, particularly with superficial stroking.	McMillan's technique of maintaining contact on the return stroke is being used by most operators.
17. Do you ever "stroke off" a whole area, such as the back, the upper extremity, or the lower extremity?	No description of such a technique can be found in Hoffa's text.	The back is stroked off when each division has been effleuraged and on the forearm as a final stroke.	Mennell's "superficial stroking" is similar but of a superficial nature only.	McMillan's influence has been felt in that the majority use this technique.

USE OF THE VARIOUS STROKES

QUESTION	HOFFA	McMILLAN	MENNELL	CONCLUSIONS FROM QUESTIONNAIRE RESULTS
1. Which of the effleurage strokes are used?	Hoffa describes the use of: Light and deep stroking Knuckling Circular effleurage Thumb stroking Alternate-thumb stroking Simultaneous stroking.	McMillan describes the use of: Light and deep stroking Simultaneous stroking Alternate-hand stroking.	Mennell describes the use of: Superficial stroking Deep effleurage Simultaneous stroking.	The majority of the operators use an effleurage that is predominantly the same, light and deep stroking, and simultaneous stroking. Alternate-hand stroking, which was mentioned by McMillan is widely used as well as one-hand-over-the-other for deeper pressure. Also of note is the tendency for the operator to pick up Mennell's idea of superficial stroking, although they do not do it in the prescribed manner.
2. Which of the petrissage strokes are used?	Hoffa describes the use of petrissage which is: One-handed Two-handed (with flat hand for large flat surfaces and pick-up where possible) Two-fingered.	McMillan describes the use of petrissage which is: One-handed Two-handed With alternate hands Finger and thumb For small areas Flat-handed on the back.	Mennell describes use of: Kneading (circular movements in opposite directions) Petrissage (raising muscle mass away from subjacent tissues) One-handed.	Hoffa's techniques for petrissage are predominantly in use; McMillan's two-hand petrissage and Mennell's are very similar and this stroke is used by some.

Question	Hoffa	McMillan	Mennell	Conclusions from Questionnaire Results
3. Which of the friction strokes are used?	Hoffa describes the use of friction which uses: The thumb The index finger Both thumb and index finger.	McMillan describes the use of friction which uses: The thumb Two or three fingers The thenar eminence.	Mennell describes friction which uses any part of the hand, but especially the tips of the fingers or the balls of the thumbs.	Use of the heel of the hand and one-over-the-other for pressure are not described by any of the basic texts, but are being used widely. Other techniques concerning friction are predominantly the same, except for the few people who combine friction and petrissage into a stroke which resembles both strokes.
4. a. Is tapotement used routinely? b. Which of the tapotement strokes are used?	a. Tapotement is used routinely. b. Hacking is the only tapotement stroke that is described.	a. McMillan describes the use of tapotement routinely for a general massage. b. Tapotement strokes described are: Hacking Clapping Tapping Beating.	a. Mennell describes the use of tapotement but does not use it routinely. b. He describes the use of: Hacking Clapping Beating.	a. Whereas Hoffa used tapotement routinely and McMillan described its use in a general massage, Mennell states that he does not use it routinely and the majority of the people surveyed use it for certain pathological conditions only. b. Use of the various strokes is fairly unified.

247

QUESTION	HOFFA	McMILLAN	MENNELL	CONCLUSIONS FROM QUESTIONNAIRE RESULTS
5. How is vibration used?	Hoffa does vibration either with the points of the fingers or with a flat hand but advises the use of a mechanical vibrator.	McMillan describes vibration as being done with one finger or several and also with the flat hand.	Mennell believes that the hand is a poor substitute for a mechanical vibrator.	Although described by all three of the basic texts, it is used very little.
6. Which other strokes are used?	None.	The five fundamental procedures can form the basis for a large variety of manipulations.	Mennell describes "shaking" in which the hand grasps the part giving quick firm vibrations which shake it from side to side. He also mentions a stroke which is similar to friction, but it is applied in a transverse plane to the muscle fibers.	Horizontal stroking for the low back is rather widely used although very few have a name for this stroke. Mennell's frictionlike stroke, which is done in a transverse plane, is used by some. Although used by only a few, Storms' technique for nodules has made some impression in this country.

Suggestions for Practical Testing

Applications of massage techniques are difficult to evaluate, and grades are often subjective. Since people have the right to as accurate an evaluation as possible, the following chart is suggested as a means to a numerical evaluation on which a grade can be given. Apparent weaknesses can also be noted.

With this form the instructor can list an entire class on one page, making possible a comparison of all marks. There are 24 items to evaluate, each of which can be given a maximum score of 4. This gives a numerical total of 96 and allows 4 points which can be subtracted or added under "remarks" for incidentals not listed among the other 24. These could be such things as "leaning on the patient," or "dragging a towel or sleeve across the part to be treated."

In this way the instructor can justify the grade by showing a numerical mark. The form also provides a written record which can be reviewed with the operator.

Some instructors may prefer a briefer form. Table A-2 is a form that can be used for one person. This leaves more room for remarks than the one previously shown. It can also be evaluated numerically.

Practical Evaluation Sheet for Instructor's Use in Massage

Name _____

Statement of Problem or Case:

	GRADE	REMARKS
+10 Positioning		
+10 Draping		
+10 Choice and Use of Lubricant		
+20 Organization Overall Approach		
+20 Skill in Technique		
+10 Termination Dressing, etc.		
+20 Overall Impression		
Final Grade		

Practical Evaluation Sheet for Instructor's Use in Massage

Technique of Operator	Name of Operator									
Draping										
Positioning										
Effleurage, Rhythm										
" Pressure										
" Pattern										
Petrissage, Rhythm										
" Pressure										
" Progression										
Friction, Rhythm										
" Pressure										
" Pattern										
Tapotement, Rhythm										
" Pressure										
" Pattern										
Vibration										
Other Strokes										
Use of Lubricant										
Posture										
Condition of Hands										
Personal Appearance										
Knowledge of Case										
Attitude, Poise										
Overall Approach										
Clean-Up										
Remarks										
Numerical Total										
Final Grade										

GRADING KEY
A—Excellent   4
B—Above Average   3
C—Average   2
D—Below Average 1
F—Failing   0

Remarks

Bibliography

Academy of Traditional Chinese Medicine. *An Outline of Chinese Acupuncture*. Peking: Foreign Language Press, 1975.

Cousins, Norman. "Anatomy of an Illness (as Perceived by the Patient)," *Saturday Review*. May 28, 1977, pp. 4-6, 48-51.

Cyriax, James, *Textbook of Orthopaedic Medicine*, Vol. II, 9th ed. London: Ballière Tindall, 1977.

Dicke, Elisabeth. *Meine Bindegewebsmassage*. Stuttgart: Hippokrates-Verlag, 1956.

Downing, George. *The Massage Book*. New York: Random House and Berkeley, Calif.: The Bookworks, 1974.

Ebner, M. "Peripheral Circulatory Disturbances: Treatment by Massage of Connective Tissue Reflex Zones," *Brit. J. Phys. Med.,* Vol. 19, (Aug. 1956), pp. 176-80.

Fulton, J. F. *A Text Book of Physiology*, 16th ed. Philadelphia: W. B. Saunders Co.

Goldstein, Avram, "Opioid Peptides (Endorphins) in Pituitary and Brain," *Science*, 193 (Sept. 17, 1976), pp. 1081-86.

Grad, Bernard, *et al.* "A Telekenetic Effect on Plant Growth, Part 2. Experiments Involving Treatment with Saline in Stoppered Bottles," *International Journal of Parapsychology*, 6 (1964), pp. 473-98.

Greed, Mayno. *The Healing Hand.* Cambridge, Mass.: Harvard University Press, 1975 .

Green, Elmer and Green, Alyce. "The Ins and Outs of Mind-Body Energy," *Science Year, 1974: World Book Science Annual.* Chicago, Ill.: Field Enterprises Corp., 1973.

Head, Sir Henry. *Studies in Neurology.* London: Henry Frowde and Hodder and Stoughton, 1920.

Hoffa, Albert J. *Technik der Massage,* 14th ed. Stuttgart: Ferdinand Enke, 1900.

Huang, Min Der. Medical seminar at Chinese Acupuncture Science Research Foundation, Taipei, Taiwan, R.O.C. 1975.

Ingham, Eunice D. *Stories the Feet Can Tell: Stepping to Better Health.* Rochester, N.Y.: Eunice D. Ingham, 1959.

Institute of Traditional Chinese Medicine of Hunan Province. *A Barefoot Doctor's Manual* (transl. of a Chinese Instruction to Certain Chinese Health Personnel). Washington, D.C.: U.S. Dept. of Health, Educ. & Welfare, 1974. DHEW Pub. No. (NIH) pp. 75-695.

Jacobs, M. "Massage for the Relief of Pain: Anatomical and Physiological Consideration," *Phys. Therapy Rev.,* 40:2 (Feb. 1960), pp. 96-97.

Kimber, D. C.; Gray, C. E.; Stackpole, C. E.; Leavell, L. C. *Textbook of Anatomy and Physiology,* 14th ed. New York: The Macmillan Company, 1961.

Krieger, Dolores. "Nursing Research for a New Age," *Nursing Times,* (April 1976), pp. 1-7.

Krieger, Dolores. "The Relationship of Touch with Intent to Help or Heal, to *Ss* In-vivo Hemoglobin Valves: A Study in Personalized Interactions," *Proc. American Nurses Assoc. 9th Nursing Research Conference.* Kansas City: The Assoc., 1973.

Marx, Jean L. "Neurobiology: Researchers High on Endogenous Opiates," *Science,* 193 (Sept. 24, 1976), pp. 1227-28.

McGarey, William A. *Acupuncture and Body Energies.* Phoenix, Ariz.: Gabriel Press, 1974.

McMillan, Mary. *Massage and Therapeutic Exercise,* 3rd ed. Philadelphia: W. B. Saunders Co., 1932.

Mennell, James B. *Physical Treatment by Movement, Manipulation, and Massage,* 5th ed. Philadelphia: The Blakiston Co., and London: J. A. Churchill, Ltd., 1945.

Namikoshi, Tokujiro. *Shiatsu: Health & Vitality at Your Fingertips.* San Francisco: Japan Publications, Inc., 1969.

Ohashi, Wataru. *Do It Yourself Shiatsu.* Toronto: Clark Irwin & Co., 1976.

Rice, Ruth D. "Premature Infants Respond to Sensory Stimulation," *American Psychological Assoc. Monitor,* 6:11 (Nov. 1975), pp. 8-9.

Rogers, P. A. M. "Enkephalins," *Acupuncture Research Quarterly,* 1:2 (April 1977), p. 64.

Serizawa, Katsusuke. *Massage: The Oriental Method.* San Francisco, Calif.: Japan Publications, Inc., 1974.

Stanford Univ. Medical Center, "The Morphine Within," *The Healing Arts,* 7:1 (1977), pp. 7-8.

Storms, H. D. "Diagnostic and Therapeutic Massage," *Arch. Phys. Med.,* 25 (Sept. 1944), pp. 550-52.

Tompkins, Peter, and Bird, Christopher. *The Secret Life of Plants.* New York: Avon, 1973.

Tsay, Robert C. *Textbook of Chinese Acupuncture Medicine, Vol. I, General Introduction to Acupuncture.* Wappingers Falls, N.Y. and Las Vegas, Nev.: Assoc. of New Chinese Medicine and East-West Medical Center, Ltd., 1974.

Wang, Julie. "Breaking Out of the Pain Trap," *Psychology Today,* 11:2 (July 1977), pp. 78-82, 86.

References—Acupuncture

Academy of Traditional Chinese Medicine. *An Outline of Chinese Acupuncture.* Peking: Foreign Language Press, 1975.

Beau, Georges. *Chinese Medicine,* New York: Avon Books. The Hearst Corporation, 1972.

Chan, Pedro. *Wonders of Chinese Acupuncture,* Alhambra, California: Borden Publishing Co., 1973.

Duke, Marc. *Acupuncture,* New York: Pyramid House, 1972.

Hashimoto, Mme. Dr. M. *Japanese Acupuncture,* New York: Liveright Publishing Corp., 1968.

Huard, Pierre and Wong, Ming. *Chinese Medicine,* New York: World University Library, McGraw-Hill Book Co., 1968.

John E. Fogarty International Center. "Acupuncture Anesthesia" CA Translation of a Chinese Publication of the same title, DHEW Publication No. (NIH) 75-785, 1975.

Kao, F. F. and Kao J. J. "Acupuncture Therapeutics: An Introductory Text." A compilation and translation by F. F. Kao, New Haven: Eastern Press, 1973.

Manaka, Yoshio and Urquharth, Ian A. *The Layman's Guide to Acupuncture,* New York: John Westerhill, Inc., 1972.

Mann, Felix. *Acupuncture, the Ancient Chinese Art of Healing,* New York: Vintage Books, Random House, Inc., 1973.

Mann, Felix. *Atlas of Acupuncture, Points and Meridians in Relation to Surface Anatomy,* London: William Heinemann Medical Books, Ltd., 1966.

Mann, Felix. *The Treatment of Disease by Acupuncture,* London: William Heinemann Medical Books, Ltd., 1967.

Palos, Stephan. *The Chinese Art of Healing,* New York: Bantam Books, Inc., 1972.

Tan, L. T., Tan, M. Y.-C., and Veith, I. *Acupuncture Therapy: Current Chinese Practice,* Philadelphia: Temple University Press, 1973.

Wallnofer, Heinrich and Von Rottausher, Anna. *Chinese Folk Medicine,* New York: Signet Books, 1972.

Veith, Ilza. *The Yellow Emperor's Classic of Internal Medicine,* University of California Press, 1972.

Wei-P'Ing, Wu. *Chinese Acupuncture,* Translated from Chinese to French by J. Lauier; to English from French by Philip M. Chancellor. Rustington, Sussex, England: Health Sciences Press, 1962.

Worsley, J. R. *Is Acupuncture for You?,* New York: Harper & Row, 1972.

JOURNALS

The American Journal of Chinese Medicine. Garden City, New York.

Index

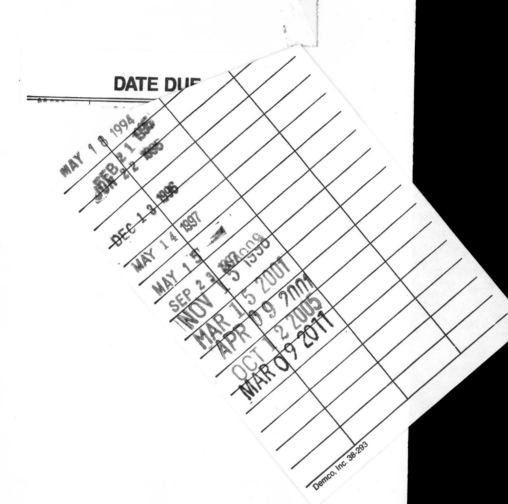

DATE DUE

MAY 1 8 1994
FEB 2 1 1995
JUN 2 2 1995
DEC 1 3 1995
DEC 1 4 1997
MAY 1 4 1997
MAY 1 1998
SEP 2 3 1999
NOV 1 5 2001
MAR 1 5 2001
APR 0 9 2001
OCT 1 2 2005
MAR 0 9 2011

Demco, Inc. 38-293